GETTING

Veterinary School

FOURTH EDITION

JAMES BURNETT

TROTMAN

GW01036093

This fourth edition published in 2003 in Great Britain
by Trotman and Company Ltd
2 The Green, Richmond, Surrey TW9 1PL

© Trotman and Company Ltd 2003

First edition published in 1995, second edition published in 1999, by Trotman
and Company Ltd, author John Handley, third edition published in 2001

British Library Cataloguing in Publication Data
A catalogue record for this book is available from the British Library

ISBN 0 85660 862 9

Typeset by Mac Style Ltd, Scarborough
Printed and bound in Great Britain by Creative Print & Design (Wales) Ltd

CONTENTS

For up-to-date information on veterinary schools go to
www.mpw.co.uk/getintomed

ACKNOWLEDGEMENTS

The additional information contained in the fourth edition of Getting into Veterinary School was researched by Fiona Munro. I would like to thank her, Emma Godwin who allowed me to use her UCAS Personal Statement, all of the people who contributed to the previous editions of this book, the staff and students at the six UK veterinary schools, UCAS and the RCVS. I am grateful to the veterinary practitioners and students who gave up their time to answer my questions.

INTRODUCING THE ISSUES

In 2001, 1613 people applied for entry to veterinary school, about the same number as in the previous two years. Of these, 702 were accepted, a success rate of about 44%. For potential vets, the most important question is 'What can I do to make sure that I am in that 44% when I apply?' The aim of this book is to give you that information. However, there is no secret formula that will ensure success. The students who are accepted work hard to gain their places. They are motivated and determined, and their desire to work within the field of veterinary science is deep-rooted and genuine. Having said that, even the most promising candidate will not get a place if he or she does not prepare properly.

This book *is* about getting into veterinary school, it is *not* about giving up and trying something else. The tone is a balanced mixture of realism and optimism. Yes, there is cause for hope despite the undeniable fact that getting into veterinary school is extremely difficult, given the competition for places. No one should minimise the hard road that lies ahead. Getting into one of the six veterinary schools in the UK is just the first stage on the route to becoming a qualified veterinary surgeon with all the inevitable hard work and dedication that follows. The key to success lies within each individual. That is what this book is all about.

The motivational factor

Academic ability is absolutely necessary. Unless there is clear potential for science in the sixth form this book alone cannot help. Students attracted towards veterinary science should have a natural academic ability in the sciences. If that ability spells out a confident prediction of high grades at A-level that will be a great help but even that will not be enough on its own to get into one of the veterinary schools. Applicants have to show proof of their interest, enthusiasm and commitment. They have to provide evidence that they really do want to become vets.

Those slightly less academically gifted can take heart from this. High A-level performance can be attained if it is coupled with strong motivation. This is not something which derives from pep talks, but the kind of inner motivation and self-belief that spurs you on to greater efforts. This is because deep in your heart you do really want to become a vet, so much so that you are prepared to make the necessary sacrifices in terms of perseverance and effort.

Taking a practical view

This is a practical book aimed at helping someone in this situation. The competition for entry to veterinary school is tough, but the evidence in this book will show that the prospect is not so daunting that it should put off someone who is keen, practical and intelligent. So how do you know that this is the career for you and that you are not wasting your own and everyone else's time? These are some of the questions addressed in this book.

A top priority must be to become so well informed and acquainted with the work of a vet that you know that you have made the right choice of career. What are the factors involved in course choice? Have you considered all of them? What do the courses have in common? What are the factors that influence the admissions tutors to come down in favour of one well-qualified candidate against another? What happens at interview? What about the various career choices open to the newly qualified vet? How are the country's 13,000 or so qualified and economically active vets distributed in the different branches of the profession?

Personal qualities

What do customers who use the services of veterinary surgeons look for in a 'good' vet? Does this sound like the kind of profession that would suit you? Putting academic skill on one side for a moment, would you feel comfortable dealing with your customers as well as the animals? The first thing you learn in veterinary practice is that every animal brings an owner with them. How would you handle a sceptical dalesman or a 'townie' anxious and watchful as you come into contact with their beloved pet? Animals play a crucial part in the lives of their owners and

2

whether the vet handles this with tact and understanding will be the deciding factor in both their professional and personal development.

Facing up to controversy

Controversy is no stranger to the veterinary profession. Progress in the shape of new techniques, vaccines and medicines no longer meets the resistance that it once did. Preventive medicine has saved a lot of lives through mass vaccination or treating deficiencies through the feed. However, other time-honoured controversies persist. For example, even among vets, views differ about the virtues of vegetarianism. Fox hunting also has its devotees as well as its detractors. What do you feel about trying to rear a new type of animal? Do you have a problem with rearing animals for wool or meat? What about rearing animals to supply organs for humans? What are your views? Do you have a view? What would you have to say if you were called for interview and asked these kinds of questions? True to its practical aims this book will draw attention to ways in which you might respond.

Who will find this book helpful?

This book is intended to help all those attracted to the veterinary profession because of their strong interest in animals and their sympathy and respect for them, which is both caring and scientific. They must have the ability and intention to study science A-levels (or their equivalent). *Furthermore, they must combine practical ability with the scientific interest and an interest in people.*

Those charged with the responsibility of helping students make these important decisions about their future, careers teachers and careers officers in particular, will find this book helpful as will parents anxious to assist their son or daughter.

This book may also help to put off those who feel drawn towards animals for mainly sentimental reasons. They may come to realise that they would not cope so well with the owners – who willingly pay the full cost of the vet's services out of their own pocket because their pet means so much to them. No matter how good you are you've failed unless you can get your message across to the owner so that the animal gets the right treatment.

3

Student views

A feature of this book is the presence of the student view. Those who are now undergraduates on veterinary courses said that they would have appreciated knowing the views of people in their position when they were at school. Often panels made up of students returning to their former schools to give careers advice do not include a veterinary student. This book therefore includes several student profiles.

For up-to-date information on veterinary schools go to
www.mpw.co.uk/getintomed

COMMITMENT

Wanting to become a veterinary surgeon is one of life's medium-term aims. It requires perseverance and a lot of determination. If all goes well and you get the kind of sixth form science results demanded by all the veterinary schools, it will still take a further five or six years to qualify. Most people faced with the need for intensive study in the sixth form will find it hard to look further ahead than the next test or practical. Yet much more than this is needed if you are to stand a chance of getting into vet school. Ideally the pursuit of this interest in animals and their welfare should have started much earlier. There are numerous cases of aspiring vets who have begun their enquiries as early as the age of 12, and certainly many have started gaining their practical experience by the age of 14.

Some vets have grown up on a farm and knew that they wanted this kind of life. Others have come from an urban background and have developed an interest despite some not inconsiderable environmental difficulties. This can be started in a variety of ways and can develop through, for instance, pet ownership, the Herriot books, one of the numerous TV programmes like *Vets in Practice*, or the influence of a friend. 'It's a great life, there's so much variety,' was one student's view. 'You realise it when you start going out getting experience. You see that you can be a vet in a town or in the countryside, that some practices are much larger than others and that some are very busy while others appear more relaxed.'

One young vet told me that she had begun her enquiries at about the age of 14 and started working at weekends. Her experience began with work in kennels, a dairy farm and a stables where she began to learn horse riding.

Strong interest

An interest in animals and their welfare is fundamental. *'The veterinary profession has an important role to play in providing advice and treatment for the nation's pets, in maintaining the health and welfare of the nation's herds and flocks and in safeguarding public health.'* This is the view of the Royal College of Veterinary Surgeons.

The interest must be wholehearted but not sentimental or just concerned with cuddly animals. 'It's not just a matter of loving animals,' says Norman Henry, an experienced Cheshire veterinary surgeon. 'You must love to work with them; that's a big difference.' Most vets enjoy their job because it enables them to seek a treatment that will work and they love it when they see an improvement in the cow, horse, poodle, rabbit, and all the others they treat.

After you qualify as a veterinary surgeon you are admitted as a member of the Royal College of Veterinary Surgeons, status which confers upon you the right to practise in member states of the European Union. The College will admit you to the Register in a short ceremony in the course of which you have to solemnly declare 'that my constant endeavour will be to ensure the welfare of animals committed to my care.' This means that once you are admitted you have the legal right to practise veterinary surgery on all animals under all conditions.

Professional commitment

It follows that your training will have prepared you to deal with all aspects of the work. You will have attended the inspection of animals slaughtered for meat production. Every person training to be a veterinary surgeon has to spend a week in an abattoir; this is a compulsory requirement of the course.

Further, you may not have thought about the use of animals in the teaching programme. It is generally kept to a minimum and it is increasingly video-based, but you must be prepared to take part in practical classes in which animal tissues are handled or used. All veterinary schools show concern and respect for animals and stress the importance of this at all stages in the undergraduate programme. In short, your training will have prepared you in all aspects of veterinary science so that you can undertake to treat all animals whether they are reared for food, used/kept for laboratory research or as pets. This is what is meant by an unsentimental attachment to animal welfare.

Animal welfare comes first at all times; this is a basic professional commitment. However, if you have anti-vivisectionist beliefs and are not prepared to undertake practical work as a professional, you will not get into veterinary school. It would be better for you to consider putting your scientific interest and ability to other uses. This may seem unfair but it is absolutely essential that the prospective candidate realises that no veterinary student can claim exemption on conscientious grounds from any part of the training.

Why practical experience is so important

Confirmation of a period spent at a veterinary establishment is one of the conditions for entry to an undergraduate course leading to the degree of Bachelor of Veterinary Medicine or Science. Some might think that is a conclusive argument for getting practical experience, but there is more to it than that.

Without getting out and finding what it is like to deal with normal, healthy animals as well as sick ones, how will you know that you are suited to a career dedicated to providing a service to animals and their owners? As one student put it, 'Knowing what animals look like doesn't necessarily prepare you for what it feels or smells like. There's only one way to find out and that is to get into close contact.' You may think you love animals because of the way you feel about your own pet, but going from the particular to the general may cause you to think quite differently. So check it out, you might even be allergic to some animals. Make certain that you still feel happy about dealing with animals in general and really mean business.

Work experience is also vital if you are to have a chance of being called for interview, and without an interview you cannot be offered a place. Some of the veterinary schools are more specific than others about what they expect in the way of practical experience. The Royal Veterinary College, for example, specifies 'at least six weeks "hands on" experience: two weeks with one or more veterinary practices; two weeks or more working with larger domestic animals on a livestock farm; and two weeks of other animal experience (eg kennels, riding school, zoo etc.)'. Cambridge is more relaxed about work experience. The Cambridge website states that 'it is helpful to have some personal experience of the veterinary profession and have a realistic idea what the work may entail. However, extensive experience is not a prerequisite and seeing a variety of different aspects of the profession for relatively short periods can be more helpful.' Glasgow advises applicants that 'experience working with veterinarians so that the applicant has some understanding of the duties and responsibilities of a practitioner, is essential before making such a career choice.'

One way to start

Go to a cattery or the local riding stables or kennels and see healthy animals as an early move. One student told me that she had done kennel work at weekends for four years before becoming a veterinary student. Cleaning out kennels is a dirty, often unpleasant job and to do this over such a long period shows dedication. This is the way to demonstrate commitment.

Follow up a visit to the local cattery or kennels with at least a week with your local vet and then see how you feel. The point is that you are not just trying to satisfy the admissions tutors at veterinary school, important though that is, you are testing your own motivation. This is vital, for make no mistake, you are going to need all the focus you can muster. The task you are about to set yourself is going to draw upon all your dedication and determination.

Making the initial contact

Some vets express reluctance to allow young inexperienced people into their practice. This is understandable. They know that many people are attracted by the idea of becoming a vet; they have, after all, seen many TV programmes! Look at this from the vet's point of view. Some people are attracted to animals for emotional reasons. They may not be academically strong enough to make the grade. They may be so impractical that they could get their finger nipped through one of the animal cages in the first half hour. 'They do need to have manual skills,' noted one vet. 'They do need to be able to tie their own shoelaces!' So why should the vet end up wasting his or her time?

Don't be surprised if some vets suggest that you should first visit for just a day. The reason for this is that they feel they need to meet you first before committing themselves. As one vet said, 'You can get a fair idea in the first few hours; some are bright and a pleasure to have around.'

Making the initial contact can also be quite difficult for a student, often because of the nervous inexperience of the caller or because the vet is cautious and reluctant to take on an unknown commitment. This is where parents can help. If a parent knows that their son or daughter is serious and is showing promise at school in the sciences, they can be a real help by speaking to the vet and giving reassurance. Generally vets will react favourably to a parent's call because it means that the contact is serious. Once the initial opening has been made the ensuing development of contacts is best left to the student as part of their growing self-reliance.

Your local vet will know a lot of people through working with animals. A recommendation, or better still an introduction of yourself by your local vet to a large animal practice or a local farmer, may lead to work in a stables or work with sheep. You get to know people yourself and this builds your confidence. Developing contacts in this way is known as 'networking'.

Gaining experience

What will the local vet ask you to do? This will depend upon the vet. 'We cannot afford to waste time so we begin by asking about their capability for science A-levels at grades A and B,' remarked one vet. 'We give them three days of blood and gore to see what it's all about. In our case, they will see a farm. We insist on wellies and a good standard of dress, no jeans or open-necked shirts!' Alternatively, your local vet may be a small practice dealing mainly with companion animals, ie most often cats and dogs, but also rabbits, goldfish, gerbils and budgies. Some students may themselves have gained experience breeding bantams, ferrets, pigeons or fish. This all points to a strong interest.

Some practices are mixed, dealing with farm animals, horses and pets, while in country areas there are practices that deal mainly with farm animals. The type of practice and its size varies widely. The average practice has three or four vets, while at the one extreme about 2% have more than 10 with a degree of specialisation; others, about one in four, are single-handed, requiring practitioners to deal with a wide range of work. This being so, the resources that the vet will be able to draw upon will also vary widely.

Small animals

A student who is still at school or college will be fortunate indeed to find themselves in the consulting room with the vet. This is because anxious owners will not always appreciate or understand the need for someone of school age to be present. It is much more likely that you will be asked to spend time with the veterinary nurses. As one vet commented, 'Let's see if they can handle animals. Are they frightened?' The idea is to see how the student reacts to aspects of animal husbandry at an early stage. If they cannot abide cleaning up the blood and faeces that goes with animal practice then they should in all probability seek out another career and save themselves and others a lot of wasted time. After an artery has stopped pumping or diarrhoea has ended, there is a clean-up job to be done and that is an early experience for many well-intentioned potential vets. Can they take it?

A head nurse in a medium-sized mixed practice listed six headings under which they observe how students helping in the small-animal surgery are shaping up. This is what she told me:

- How keen are they to help in every area? For example do they clean up willingly?
- How observant are they? Do they watch how we do the bandaging or how we hold the animal straight ready for an injection? Do they watch carefully how we take a blood sample, administer an anaesthetic or set up an intravenous drip?
- Do they maintain a neat and tidy appearance and clean themselves up before going in to see a small-animal client? This is very important to the owner.
- Are they friendly towards the client, do they make conversation and try to establish a relationship?
- Do they ask questions about what they don't understand? They shouldn't be afraid to ask even while procedures are being carried out.
- Is the student listening to what is being said and the way it is being said? Do they appreciate the experience that allows the vet to counsel owners on sensitive issues? For example, on reducing their favourite

pet's diet. This is not an easy message to get across to an over-indulgent owner and it needs a good bedside manner for the vet to be able to tell the owner what must be done without giving offence.

Working on the farm

Some students have the chance to gain early experience on a nearby farm. Make contact yourself or try asking your local vet for an introduction. What would you do? One farmer's wife commented, 'We would expect a 14-year-old to help feed the livestock, to help with bedding-up, ie putting fresh straw in the pens and sweeping up.' You should be alert to what is happening around you. Before long you may start asking questions: 'Why is that calf coughing? What are you giving it?'

If you are still interested and return for more you will be taken more seriously by the practice. This is the opportunity to get used to handling animals and thereby learning how to control them. You begin to see the normal way in which animals are housed and fed. In doing so you will gain insight into the way animals are treated and their part in the economy. You will appreciate that in many cases the animals are required for food and will ultimately be sent for slaughter, while others like horses are more akin to pets. Eventually the chance will come to go out with the vet on his or her visits to assist. This is when you learn how to hold animals, for example at lambing time.

One student told me how he recalled having to help keep hold of the animals during tuberculin testing in the midst of driving rain while calling out numbers. The way he told it you felt that he regarded that experience as his reward! This is the kind of help that the busy vet remembers when the time comes for a reference.

The importance of self-reliance

Taking the initiative like this can do you more favours than always relying on the careers department at your school. However, it is worth checking to see whether your school careers department can help you. Frankly, some school careers departments are much better organised than others. If the careers programme is well organised and planned on an established contact basis it would be sensible to enlist the department's help. However, do bear in mind that there is concern among some vets that placements organised by schools are not always carefully matched. If you have any doubts on this score you will be well advised to take the initiative in making your own arrangements. Remember that in the end it is your own responsibility to get practical experience. Busy people like vets and farmers are likely to be more impressed with those who exhibit the confidence and self-reliance to make their own approaches.

Checklist of things you can do

Always take up any opportunities that you are offered. It is variety of experience that will not only broaden your understanding of the profession you seek to join, but will also impress the admissions tutors when they come to scrutinise your UCAS form. Here are some suggestions.

- Try to get work experience in catteries and/or boarding kennels.
- Try working in the local pet shop.
- Make contact with a local vet and indicate your interest by helping with some of the menial tasks. If you are keen you will not mind the dirty work.
- Aim to get at least two to three weeks' experience with a large-animal veterinary practice or occasional days or weekends over a long period. Without this you will not be taken into veterinary school no matter how well qualified you are academically. You must also gain some experience of working in a companion animal practice. Some candidates are fortunate in having access to mixed practices in which they can gain familiarity with handling large and small animals.
- Visit a local dairy farm and get acquainted with farmwork, which accounts for at least 30% of all veterinary science work. Try also to assist on a sheep farm at lambing time.
- Endeavour to get experience working with horses at a riding stables. (Remember that riding establishments are subject to inspection by an authorised veterinary surgeon.)
- Arrange to visit an abattoir if possible.
- Look into the possibility of making contact with one of the animal charities, such as the People's Dispensary for Sick Animals (PDSA) or the Royal Society for the Prevention of Cruelty to Animals (RSPCA), and find out about their work.

- Do not ignore the chance to spend a day in a pharmaceutical laboratory concerned with the drugs used by vets as well as medics or a laboratory of the Department for Environment, Food and Rural Affairs (Defra).
- Try for any additional relevant experience that may be within your reach, eg at a zoo, where you could work as an assistant to a keeper, or in a safari or wildlife park.
- Make a point of visiting local racecourses and greyhound tracks, paying particular attention to how the animals are treated. Maybe your local vet has a part-time appointment to treat the horses or dogs. If the offer comes to visit with the vet you should take it.
- Visit country events like point-to-point races, even if it is only to see what goes on. One day you may get an admissions interview and the more you know about what happens to animals in different situations the better.

Variety of experience

It cannot be emphasised too strongly that it is the *variety* of your experience that is important rather than solely its duration. A visit of just one day to a different veterinary practice where you watched small animal work, followed by another visit to a mixed practice where you were able to see a surgical procedure carried out will be impressive, particularly if you can combine this with stables work, some contact with local farms and at least some experience in, for instance, a set of kennels. If you can demonstrate convincing commitment to one or two of the local professionals there is no doubt that this will count strongly in your favour when the competition for places in vet school is at its fiercest.

What will impress people is the fact that you have willingly returned to your local vet's practice over a period of time and only the vet will know what it has cost you to do this. True, you have seen lots of interesting and varied activities and met many interesting people, but the truth is that many of your friends would have melted away had they been asked and expected to do what you have had to do. Let's face it, not many students would have returned to the practice after having to clean up and deal with blood and muck time and again.

It's vital to get as much experience as you possibly can for two important reasons.

- It proves that you know that you do really want to become a vet.
- The veterinary school wants you to be certain and will look for the evidence.

Gaining practical experience is crucial in your endeavour to get into veterinary school and, because of its part in getting you focused on your ultimate objective, to become a member of the Royal College of Veterinary Surgeons.

STUDENT PROFILE

Colin's family lived in London for the first 15 years of his life before moving to Norfolk. Colin, now 21 years old, still lives in London and is completing his third year of study.

'I suppose I've known that I wanted to be a vet from about the age of 12–13 years old when I first became aware of the job through the Herriot books, as I had never had a pet and lived in central London. Since then I've seen quite a lot of what the job entails and the challenge, interest and variety of the job appeals strongly.

'I began by calling on a local practice in Norfolk and was told to come back at 15. I did so and soon struck up a friendship with one of the partners with whom I have since seen most of my practice, and who has helped set up additional experiences during weekends and holidays. For example, about a week each at a cattle farm, horse stables, kennels and a cattery.

'I was quite relaxed over my A-levels as quite frankly I didn't really believe I would get AAB first time. As I'd done AS-level Maths in my fifth year and didn't want to do Physics, my choice was to do Biology, Chemistry and Maths. I think avoiding stress and worry is most important, as well as practising questions rather than note-reading. In the event I surprised mysef with two A grades and a B in Maths.

'To survive on the veterinary science course you should be good at managing your work, my weakest point! There are a lot of social events organised, and it can be hard to "work, rest and play" in the right order. Time management includes organising work experience during the vacations. This can be hard, as I'm quite likely to be retaking some exams.

'The course is hard work. There's a lot to learn that doesn't always seem very relevant, especially in the first two years, but the more practically relevant it gets, the better. And there is the goal at the end – the idea of joining a profession that represents a way of life and a worthwhile career.'

WHAT MAKES A GOOD VET?

This question is at the heart of the matter because it is a career aim that calls for considerable sacrifice in terms of time and effort. Certainly every veterinary practice has to organise itself so that someone is on call 24 hours a day for 365 days a year. As one farmer commented, 'A vet needs to have a darn good sense of humour to be called out at 3am on a cold night to deal with a difficult calving and having to get down in six inches of muck!' It is certainly not a career for someone lacking in confidence, or who holds back and carries an air of uncertainty. A good vet will be able to diagnose most things, 'but if you can't,' says Norman Henry, 'it's your job to know who can. The secret is to know your own limitations.' This is particularly important for the newly qualified veterinary surgeon. 'New vets,' according to experienced Cheshire farmer, David Faulkner, 'must know when to seek help and be mature enough not to be too embarrassed for there are always a lot of new things still to learn.'

The farmer's view

'Farmers know immediately if they are going to get on with you,' an experienced vet revealed. 'They look at the way you handle and approach the animals. If you can't catch 'em the owner will lose confidence and you won't be allowed anywhere near the livestock.' A seasoned farmer confided, 'Give me a vet who doesn't wait to be asked and is out giving you a hand.' He added, 'If they are confident in what they are doing it soon comes across.' Farmers and animal owners generally like to have a vet who communicates well, has a sense of humour, is outgoing rather than shy and reserved, and is able to walk into any situation and have an answer.

Prevention

A recent poll showed that vets are still held in high esteem by the general public. The popular image of a vet is of someone working long hours, who's able and caring, whose charges are not too high and who doesn't worry too much about bills being paid promptly! People also pictured vets driving around at breakneck speed with a briefcase and a big bag of drugs – the traditional image of the fire brigade service.

Today there's a lot of knowledge about preventive health by diet and vaccination. Whole herds can be treated at the right time of year. Farmers expect their vet to look ahead and draw their attention to that which will prevent disease – 'Look, October is approaching, why not vaccinate all the cattle and prevent pneumonia?' Feed additives can be administered in either the feed or drink. This is much better than having to go through the trauma of having to inject a whole farmyard of pigs! A good vet will seek to promote preventive medicine whenever possible. It makes sense bearing in mind that animals can't tell you they're not well. A vet can do a lot of good with vaccinations and treating deficiencies through the feed by replacing what's not there, improving not only productivity but also the welfare of the animals.

Most people will agree that prevention is better than cure but this is not always easy to achieve. Preventive medicine is costly and farmers, in particular, have a reputation of being watchful of how much they spend. There's no doubt that preventive medicine is a good investment for the future but in the aftermath of BSE, Foot and Mouth, and the collapse of much of their export market, farmers are anxious and unwilling in many cases to make the necessary outlay. Drug usage for cattle has fallen away. Often farmers don't approach the vet until there's an emergency and then you're back to the old fire brigade image of the vet rushing here and there.

In today's busy world with a general shortage of vets it's not easy to respond to this situation. I heard one experienced vet say that you should still try to take time to stop and let your eyes range over the flock or herd. 'You're not looking at all 300 or so animals, you look for the one or two animals who don't fit into the general pattern and are not looking well.'

A lot can still be done by encouraging good husbandry – by advising on the housing of the animals. A sign of a good vet is that he or she will have the latest drug information at their fingertips and will know how to treat certain conditions. Sound diplomatic advice will also be appreciated;

'Instead of my treating the animal's feet why don't you improve that footpath!'

Small animals

With farm animal practice in decline there are fewer opportunities for vets in this area so most practices are intent upon building up their small animal work. There's great variety – one moment it might be a reptile with a nutritional problem; or a cat losing weight is brought in for tests and causes the vet to wonder if there might be a problem with the animal's liver or could it be cancer? A rabbit is brought in, many are now regarded as house pets, your initial diagnosis of constipation is confirmed. Dental problems among the small-animal population occur quite frequently but obesity is also much more common than most people imagine. The vet has to counsel the owner on reducing the feed and try to gain acceptance of regular weigh-ins at the surgery.

Most of us live in a busy urban environment and a price has sometimes to be paid. It can take the form of a road accident. A dog has been hit by a vehicle and the 'crash kit' is brought out. The doses of the most commonly used drugs are marked clearly on the crash box lid, the syringes are loaded, everything is sterilised and ready. It's important to act quickly, but the true professional keeps calm; this is no time for the vet to fumble when decisive action can save the dog's life.

A good vet knows that the way the owners are dealt with is crucial because the pets mean so much to them. Unless the vet can get his or her message across the animal is not going to get the right treatment anyway. It's been truly said that the hope and trust of the owners is matched only by the trust and helplessness of the animals. To be a good vet you have to acquire that little bit extra. Imagine the scene as a 4-year-old becomes distraught when he's told that his pet hamster must be put down. How do you show empathy amid the boy's flood of tears? How do you discuss it with him? Perhaps the boy's parent will let you attempt to explain how the hamster feels and that soon the small animal's pain will cease and the end itself will not be felt. Even when you know it's the kindest thing to do, giving a lethal injection is still one of the toughest parts of the job.

So why do you want to be a vet?

A question worth asking because it is not a career that will lead to riches or glamour. So why do so many talented students find themselves attracted to the idea of becoming a vet?

Perhaps it is about adapting and fitting into a way of life. Is this what keeps everyone focused during the long hours of study? The interest in and sympathy for animals is taken for granted by many commentators, but in reality it can take the form of reacting to an emergency that puts dedication to the test. A cat is hit by a car, you know that life is slipping away, but you do your best for the distraught owner. You battle to save an animal's life in a freezing barn in the middle of the night. It's all in the vet's day or night's work and there is no one to applaud you except the grateful, or not so understanding, owner.

In James Herriot's first book, *If Only They Could Talk*, he reflects that animals are unpredictable things and that a vet's whole life is unpredictable. 'It's a long tale of little triumphs and disasters,' writes Herriot, 'and you've got to really like it to stick it ... One thing, you never get bored.' Later, on another occasion, he muses, with aching ribs and bruises all over his legs, that being a vet is, in fact, a strange way to earn a living:

'But then I might have been in an office with the windows tight shut against the petrol fumes and the traffic noise, the desk light shining on the columns of figures, my bowler hat hanging on the wall. Lazily I opened my eyes again and watched a cloud shadow riding over the face of the green hill across the valley. No, no ... I wasn't complaining.'

Some people grumble about the beguiling influence of the Herriot books. There is, however, a lot of cool reality in the pages laden with good humour and philosophy; so much so that one student described the effect of the books as leaving a 'cold afterglow'. Many professions would love to have a PR agent writing on their behalf with the skills of Herriot.

STUDENT PROFILE

Sarah studied for her A-levels at an independent school in London. Her interest in veterinary science started when she was allowed to spend a day with a vet at a small private zoo when she was 14. In the first year of A-levels, Sarah tried to organise work experience, but found it difficult since she was an accomplished sportswoman and musician, and so she had school commitments on Saturdays, as well as most evenings. The veterinary practices and animal welfare organisations that she contacted wanted volunteers to work on a regular basis, and she was unable to do so. Realising the need for work experience, Sarah looked for other opportunities:

'I managed to arrange to help out in a Riding for the Disabled centre, on Sundays, where I cleaned the stables and fed the horses. Although this was hard work, it meant that I could have contact with a local vet, who visited the stables every so often. Through him, I was able to spend a week with a friend of his, who had a practice in Dorset, and this led to my being able to spend a month on a dairy farm in the summer holidays.

'I had never regarded myself as being what you might call pushy, but I found that if I demonstrated my enthusiasm, and asked for help with a smile on my face, people were only too glad to help me. I realised that I had to try to use contacts that I had made to gain work experience if I was to succeed in convincing the vet schools that I was serious. Of course, the point of my work experience was not only to persuade the selectors but, more importantly, to prove to myself that I really wanted to be a vet.'

Sarah sat A-levels in Chemistry, Biology and Mathematics, gained AAA, and is now studying veterinary science in Scotland.

WHAT THE ADMISSIONS TUTORS SEEK

Admissions tutors try to get the best students they can for their course. That's putting it at its most basic. They are also acting in the best interests of the veterinary profession. They know that the competition is fierce and that the biggest hurdle faced by aspiring students is entry into a veterinary school. Once this obstacle is overcome there is, given the undoubted ability of those able enough to get the entry grades needed, every chance that with diligence and lots of hard work the student will in due course enter the profession. However, it is important to understand that *motivation* is the key factor in selection. It is in the last analysis more important even than A-levels or their equivalent. Therefore, the admissions tutors are looking at the total impression conveyed by the candidate on the UCAS form. This will include not only academic predictions and headteacher's report but also extracurricular interests as well as the extremely important supporting practical experience and references. In the final analysis the tutors know that they are exercising a big responsibility. Their decisions will largely shape the future profession.

TAKING A BROAD VIEW

Ideally admissions tutors will seek to have students representing a good cross-section of the community. In recent years more women are applying and being admitted than men. Then there is the question of background. Those with an upbringing in country areas can have an excellent range of experience and general knowledge of animal husbandry. Some of them may be the sons or daughters of farmers or vets. Clearly they have a lot to offer. Yet it would be unfair and divisive to fill a course with people who all had these advantages. What of the students coming from the cities where gaining practical experience is not so easy? A few places will be kept for graduates taking veterinary science as a second degree. There will also be some places reserved for overseas students who provide valuable income as well as added richness to the mix of students in all the veterinary schools. Nevertheless, the overwhelming majority of places on these courses will be filled by school-leavers or those who have taken a year out since leaving school.

Practical 'hands-on' experience

Each of the veterinary schools' admissions tutors will seek well-rounded evidence of practical experience and interest. For example, the Royal Veterinary College states that course applicants are expected to have at least six weeks of practical experience made up as follows: a minimum of two weeks with one or more veterinary practices; two weeks' experience of handling larger animals by working with farm livestock; and two weeks of other experience, eg kennels, etc. Another example is Liverpool where they want to see experience with at least three of the six main animal groups – horses, cattle, sheep, pigs, poultry and small animals. An absolute minimum of three weeks of work shadowing with vets is regarded as essential. Note that the phrases 'at least' and 'minimum' occur frequently. In other words, serious applicants should aim to do more to give themselves a chance.

Academic versus practical

Despite the strong emphasis on practical experience demanded by all the veterinary schools, many people in the veterinary profession are concerned that the high A-level grades required, currently ranging between AAA and AAB, suggests that the profession is being filled with people who, while being academically very bright, are not so hot dealing with the practical side of the work. Apart from the fact that it is often wrong to assume that academically able people are always very impractical, this worry reveals an imperfect understanding of the logistics of the UCAS (Universities and Colleges Admissions Service) operation each year and how the admissions tutors in the veterinary schools deal with it. Crucial to understanding what happens is the completion by the student of the UCAS form and the evidence of the supporting motivation.

Importance of high A-level grades and supporting motivation

Professor Gaskell, when he was Dean of Liverpool's Veterinary School, left no room for doubt that the most important thing from the admissions' point of view is the prospective student's motivation and understanding of what he or she is about. This has to come across on the student's UCAS form. This does not mean that academic ability is unimportant. There is an enormous amount that has to be learned, and Professor Gaskell advises, 'It's the same with medicine, we find that A-levels or their equivalent are good indicators of the ability to absorb, hold and recall information.'

The problem with weaker A-levels is that you may start to find the amount of learning required difficult. Fortunately veterinary science is in the position of being able to select the best of the motivated. It must be added that it is not in the interests of the profession, or the animals and their owners whom the vets serve, to relax this strong position.

Hints on getting the A-level grades

Admissions tutors will reject you for veterinary school unless you can achieve high A-level grades. This demands hard work. Most of us delay and will find excuses to put the whole thing off. Yet if you are to achieve the professional status of becoming a veterinary surgeon you just know that you are going to have to study effectively. It takes many long hours of study to get AAB or AAA. Some people will get on with their studies because of 'fear motivation' – what will my parents say if I make a mess of it? This can work for some people but how much better it is to have positive motivation. This will spur you on every time you see a good vet in action, someone you admire.

Challenge yourself to be that person. The grades sought by the veterinary schools suggest to many people that veterinary scientists are on a higher plane. The truth is that in real terms it doesn't take two As and a B to make a vet. Unfortunately the high academic standard required puts off some otherwise excellent prospective applicants. Don't be put off; if you see these grades as a means to an end, *you can do it*. Many of the students on veterinary science courses have told me that they are not specially clever, they just worked hard because they knew they had an objective and went for it. So can you. Here are ten tips to help you to do it.

1. Many sixth-formers leave things until it is too late. When you are in the lower sixth you think you have plenty of time to take time off and go partying, etc. Don't do this. Write out a weekly schedule. Know what you have to do each day.
2. Don't be too proud to ask for help from friends or teachers.
3. Set realistic goals in each subject. Your teachers can supply you with a copy of the syllabus. Where do you want to be by Christmas? By Easter?
4. Try to concentrate while studying. If you lose your focus, stop and have a complete rest and come back to it later.
5. Take your time when studying, don't try to hurry over difficult concepts.
6. Don't leave things until it is too late. When you are in year 12 you may think that you will have plenty of time to catch up later in the course. However, not only do AS results contribute 50% of the total A-level marks; but also the AS results may well be taken in to consideration by the admissions tutors when you apply.
7. Don't be too hard on yourself. We all make mistakes. When doing practice papers, remember you'll get better with each set of questions you tackle, and they help you to identify the areas you need to concentrate on.
8. Don't be afraid to experiment with study methods. Some people are better in the early morning, others prefer late at night. Some like studying to background music. Some use memory aids for formulae, etc. What works best for you?
9. Be optimistic, believe in yourself. When the going gets hard (as it inevitably will) remind yourself that it will get better. Don't forget you are going to be a member of the Royal College of Veterinary Surgeons. That is your goal.
10. Look for connections in what you are doing. A-level students gaining working experience on farms and in veterinary practice should remember that everything is related. Ask questions whenever you can, try to see the connections between subjects and whatever you are doing.

The importance of the well-rounded application

Admissions tutors in veterinary schools are faced with large numbers of candidates who are well qualified academically. To separate these applications, additional criteria have to be brought into play. This is why they attach a great deal of importance to work experience, extracurricular achievements, and the headteacher's report.

The reason for the interest attached by admissions tutors to extracurricular achievement is not hard to find. It is based upon the not unreasonable assumption that to have gained distinction in any kind of worthwhile hobby or activity demands concentration and determination. It is also an indication of the breadth of interests.

There is no reason to assume that admissions tutors in veterinary schools are any different from others in preferring students who are going to bring into college interests that will enliven and enrich student and college life.

The following are examples of the range of activities listed by a selection of veterinary applicants:

- qualifying as a dance instructor
- teaching dyslexic children
- playing jazz trumpet
- sporting success
- getting a sub-aqua certificate
- working in a summer camp in the USA
- Duke of Edinburgh awards
- completing an outdoor pursuits leadership course
- completing a word-processing course
- first-aid certificate
- martial-arts belt
- parachuting for charity
- helping disadvantaged children.

STUDENT PROFILE

James comes from London, and attended a state school. He was the first person in his family to have studied A-levels, and the sixth-form college that he attended had never had a veterinary science applicant before.

'I had seen a programme about vets, and I had always liked animals – my uncle kept greyhounds, and I was able to help him occasionally. However, I never really considered going to university, let alone becoming a vet, since my brothers and sisters had all left school at 16 to find jobs. However, my GCSE Biology teacher encouraged me, and the local careers office helped me to choose the right A-levels.

'I had to get a part-time job in the local supermarket, working evenings and weekends, in order to support myself, and my opportunities for animal-related work experience were limited. I went to open days and talked to admissions tutors who were very encouraging. I was able to shadow a vet who worked at race tracks and greyhound meetings, and he was able to give me help in writing the personal statement on the UCAS form. My careers teacher wrote my reference and explained that it had been difficult to gain more work experience and I think that the vet schools must have taken this into account because I got two interviews.

'The first one went really badly – I had never had an interview before, and I was nervous and made the mistake of thinking that if I didn't say very much they would not be able to tell if I wasn't suitable. The second one was much better, and I was made an offer of AAB.

'Just before my A-levels, I was involved in a car accident, and spent a week in hospital. I couldn't revise properly, and I was in pain when I sat the exams. Although I was predicted AAB, I got BBC. My careers teacher rang up the vet school and explained the situation. She sent copies of my medical certificates and a letter from the hospital. The admissions tutor was very nice, but said that the grades were too low, but that if I resat Chemistry and went up from a C to an A, they would give me a place for the following year.

'I resat in January, got the A, spent the rest of the year earning money, and am now in my second year. In fact, the year out helped me in many ways. I arrived at university more mature than many of my fellow students, and was a bit more focused. The money I had saved was a great help as well, as you can imagine!'

STUDENT PROFILE

Emma applied to study veterinary science when she was studying her A-levels seven years ago. Emma went to a state school in Devon and, although she was brought up in a rural area, did not get any significant work experience while she was at school. 'It didn't really cross my mind to try to shadow any of the local vets. Some of my friends were brought up on farms and so I thought I knew enough about farming and what being a vet would be like'. Emma did well in her A-levels – she achieved A grades in Biology and Chemistry, and a B grade in Physics, but did not get any interviews. She chose instead to study Zoology, and got a place through Clearing.

During her first year she decided that she was desperate to become a vet. She spoke to the university careers advisor who told her that, whilst it was possible to get a place as a graduate, the competition was intense, and she would not get any concessions over the course length because of her Zoology degree. 'Throughout my degree course, I made sure that I got lots of work experience. I worked on farms during my holidays, and helped out at the local donkey shelter at weekends. When it came to choosing my third year project, I made sure that mine was related to veterinary science so that I could visit a local vet on a regular basis. In my third year, I applied again and this time I got an interview. I was more nervous than I had ever been in my life. The interview was longer than I expected – about half an hour, and I was absolutely grilled about my motivation. They seemed surprised that I hadn't taken a year off after my A-levels and applied again then. I explained that I only discovered that you could do that when I got to university – no one from my school ever did that. They also asked me about how I was going to fund the course. I had saved up some money from my summer jobs, and my parents had also lent me some money. I came away thinking that I had messed up the interview, but I got a letter two weeks later telling me that I had been successful. Being older than most of the other students on the course is not a problem. We all want to be vets and we work together very well. I suppose that I can handle the work load a bit better than them because I have already been through it once before.'

ENTRY TO VETERINARY SCHOOL

WHAT ARE MY CHANCES?

Although the competition increases in severity each year, the truth is that for most interested and potential applicants the chances are better than most of them or their advisers imagine. It can be off-putting to discover that fewer than one in two applicants are successful, but raw statistics do not tell the whole story. Some applicants apply without a realistic chance of being accepted because they do not have the right qualifications, have not done any investigation or work experience, or have not got either good enough GCSE grades or high enough predictions for A-level. If you discount these applicants, the likelihood of the well-motivated, well-qualified applicant receiving one or more offers increases significantly. Many potential applicants are deterred by the high academic standard, but you do not have to be extraordinarily clever to become a vet. You do have to be motivated to work extremely hard and be able to absorb a lot of information. Can you not do this if you set yourself the goal of becoming a member of the Royal College of Veterinary Surgeons?

Timing

Applications for admission to veterinary science degree courses have to be made through the Universities and Colleges Admissions Service (UCAS). Applications for veterinary science must be received by UCAS by 15 October for entry in the following year. Applications received after this may be considered by the veterinary schools, but they are not bound to do so, and given the number of applications that they will receive, it is likely that they will not do so. In order to ensure that your application reaches UCAS by the deadline, you should give the completed form to your referee at least two weeks before this date. The current UCAS application form and handbook with detailed instructions should be available free of charge from your school or college. However, if you

27

have left school, or have any difficulties in obtaining a copy, you should write after 1 July in the year preceding entry, to UCAS, Rosehill, New Barn Lane, Cheltenham, Gloucestershire GL52 3LZ.

If you wish to apply to the University of Cambridge, the blue Preliminary Application Form (PAF) can be received by the college of your choice from June onwards and must be received in Cambridge by mid-October at the latest. More information on applications to Cambridge can be found in another book in this series, *Getting into Oxford and Cambridge*. Your completed UCAS form must also be sent to the UCAS office in Cheltenham by the closing date of mid-October.

Table 1 – Applications for entry to undergraduate courses in veterinary science 2001 and 2000

	2002	2001
Home Applicants	1345	1425
Accepted	636	595
Average number of applicants per place	2.11	2.39

Accepted students (Home) by qualification 2001

	A-level	Access	BTEC/ SCOTVEC	Baccalaureate	GNVQ	Scottish Highers	Degree/ Part Degree
Accepted	466	1	8	0	2	80	69
Average number of applicants per place	2.3	2	1	–	1	1.5	1.6

Acknowledgement: UCAS Statistical Service.

Open days

It is desirable to visit the colleges that hold special interest for you on their open day. It is likely that all applicants holding a conditional offer will in any case be invited to attend, but this will vary according to timing and the policy of each university. Such a visit will give you the chance to see some of the work of the veterinary school. There will be special exhibits, possibly a video programme and most probably the chance to hear the views of the admissions tutor. There may also be the opportunity to visit the veterinary school's own field station where most of the clinical work is done in the final stages of the course, and although veterinary students are kept very busy you may get the chance to speak with some of them. Some schools actually arrange for a number of their students to accompany parties of visitors on the open day. The open day will also give you an opportunity to see the general attractions of each university as a place to live and study over the next five (or six) years.

Your school will receive details of open days with forms to be completed by those wishing to attend. If you have not heard by about a month ahead of the college open day you wish to attend, please make enquiries in your school's careers department. If you hear nothing you should take the initiative yourself and write to the school liaison office or directly to the address of the institution which interests you listed in the Appendix. You owe it to yourself to find out as much as you can. Your visit and how you felt about it could also be a talking point should you be called for interview. So don't squander the opportunity to fit one or two visits into your A-level study schedule.

If you are taking time out gaining practical experience and have already met the academic requirements, you may be able to get away to attend more open days. If this is the case you may get more than one unconditional offer and so you should certainly try to visit as many of these events as you can.

It's a good idea to make notes after each visit to an open day of your impressions and what differences you spotted. These notes will be very useful if you are called for interview when they will almost certainly ask you about your visit.

Special academic requirements for veterinary science

Every university student has to meet the general matriculation requirements of each university (consult the prospectuses) but in addition there is the special prescribed subject requirement. You should check the requirements carefully – the veterinary schools' websites carry the most up-to-date information – but it is likely that you will need three A-levels (that is, three subjects carried to A2 level), which will include Chemistry, Biology and one other science/mathematical subject. Your choice of AS and A-level subjects is vital because, whilst one veterinary school might require three sciences (including Chemistry) at AS level with two taken on to A2 level, others require Biology and Chemistry at A2, or even three sciences at A2. If you are applying to Cambridge, you should be aware that different colleges have different requirements. More details on AS and A2 levels, and on other qualifications, can be found in the chapter on Course Entry Requirements on page 42. Currently no veterinary school makes a conditional offer on three A-levels at below AAB grades. Unlike the requirements for most other courses, offers are unlikely to be made on the basis of a combination of lower sixth AS and upper sixth A-level (A2) grades, although clearly the AS grades are important because they will be stated on the UCAS form, and thus will give the admissions tutors an indication that you are on course for AAA or AAB at A-level.

What about an extra subject?

Some students have been known to query whether they should take a fifth AS-level or a fourth A-level (not including General Studies). Before doing so you should bear in mind that if you offer four A-levels your performance in all four subjects will be taken into account. So if you do feel inclined to add a fourth subject at A-level remember the high grades needed for admission (see Course Entry Requirements on page 42).

Studying outside the UK

It is possible to practise as a vet in the UK having studied overseas. The process is simpler for students who have studied in the EU, or in certain universities in Canada, Australia, South Africa or New Zealand. However, graduates from other countries can still practise in the UK if they sit and pass the Statutory Examination for Membership of the RCVS, which is held in a UK veterinary school in May/June each year. Further information for all overseas graduates can be obtained from the RCVS website – see page 85.

An option open to students who wish to study overseas, but want to undertake some of their clinical training in one of the UK veterinary schools, is the veterinary science course offered by St George's University in Grenada, West Indies. Contact details for the course can be found at the end of the book.

DEALING WITH THE UCAS FORM

The UCAS Handbook, in conjunction with the accompanying instructions on the UCAS application form, is intended to give you sufficient information to enable you to complete the form. You should also be able to consult with careers teachers and sixth-form tutors in your school. In many instances you may find that your school has available reference copies of prospectuses for individual colleges and institutions.

What follows are some suggestions on matters that require your judgement.

How many applications should I make?

You may only apply to four veterinary schools. If you apply to more than four, your UCAS form will be returned, and by the time you amend it, you may well have missed the 15 October deadline. A common question is: 'Should I put two other, non-veterinary, choices in the remaining slots?' There are arguments for and against doing so, and you will need to discuss this with your careers advisor or referee. The admissions staff at all of the veterinary schools emphasise that candidates will not be disadvantaged if they fill the remaining places with other courses. However, you should be wary of putting down courses that you are not interested in, and accepting an offer as your insurance place, since you will not be eligible for Clearing if you do so.

Therefore, holding 'insurance' offers will depend on how committed you are to veterinary science. An argument in favour of going all out for the total commitment of applying solely to veterinary schools is that if you fall short of the required grades, and have just missed out, you will almost certainly have the option of gaining entry into an alternative course through Clearing. This is because other pure and applied science courses are inevitably much less competitive and you will be able to accept an offer if you want to do so.

Which alternative courses should be listed on the UCAS form?

This is a very personal matter but something can be said on what should be avoided. You should not put down medicine or dentistry. Although veterinary science admissions tutors would not automatically exclude anyone because of this mixture, they would certainly look long and hard for overwhelming evidence that veterinary science was what you really wanted. In such circumstances you could hardly expect also to satisfy the medical admissions tutors!

All things being equal it seems logical for applications listing clearly related subjects like agriculture, equine studies, animal physiology, biochemistry, microbiology or zoology to possess that important quality of coherence and to fit in with the general thrust of your application.

Is transfer possible from another degree? What happens if I do another degree?

If you really want to become a veterinary surgeon, and with hard work you can attain the necessary academic standard, it is *not* a good idea to take a different degree. Many people are badly advised to go off and do another degree and then try and transfer from another course into veterinary science. This is not feasible because it is necessary from the beginning to study certain subjects which are exclusive to veterinary science. Examples are veterinary anatomy and ruminant physiology. Apart from which the chance of there being extra places is remote. Transfer, therefore, becomes impossible and the only way you could proceed would be to go back and start your veterinary studies at the beginning. Therefore, no one should be advised to take a different course and then try to transfer. However, it is worth noting that Cambridge has been known to make some concessions to students wishing to transfer from mainly medically related degrees. Such students might, because of the Cambridge tripos system, be able to complete a veterinary science degree at the end of six or seven years' study depending upon when the transfer was made. Note that such students will still need to study veterinary physiology and anatomy.

Further reasons why it might prove unwise to do a degree in another subject are that even if you become a graduate in another cognate subject, with an upper second, your application would be assessed on the basis of your original A-levels as well as the subsequent university study. This is done in fairness to the large number of school-leavers applying. A decisive argument for most people is that in nearly all these cases graduates in other subjects would only be admitted on a 'full cost' basis. Some colleges allocate a small number of places to graduates within the Home and EU intake. Tuition fees for these would be at full cost fees payable throughout the course. There are no scholarships available for graduate applicants.

What about deferment and taking a gap year?

The UCAS form permits you to apply at, for example, the start of your upper sixth year for entry a year after completion of your A-levels. However, you will be expected to meet the conditions of the offer in the year of application. The majority of veterinary schools now welcome students deciding to postpone their entry on to the course. The most common reasons given by students are the opportunity to travel, study or work abroad, or gain additional relevant experience for the course and profession they seek to enter. The latter reason is the one most likely to influence veterinary schools because many applicants do need to strengthen their range of relevant work experience.

You should be able to explain your plans for the year taken out. Does it involve some animal experience? Those coming from urban areas may find that undertaking a gap year of a relevant nature is more difficult to achieve. It is a good idea to discuss this matter on an informal basis with an admissions tutor and get advice.

A-level predictions

As has already been indicated, A-level performance (or its equivalent) is not a sole determinant in selection because of the importance of other motivational factors. However, the predicted A-level performance is an important factor for admissions tutors in sifting through and finding committed candidates likely to meet the stipulated academic level. Final decisions are made when the A-level results are known.

It is at this point that some rejected applicants will do better than predicted. When the admissions tutors learn that the rejected candidate has achieved top grades and is excellent in other respects, they have been known to change the original rejection to an unconditional acceptance for the *following year*. Over 100 places are settled each year in this way. Indeed, it is known that the majority of entrants to veterinary science courses will have taken a year out, whether they intended this or not.

Those whose grades slip slightly below their conditional offer will usually be considered in August and could be offered entry if places are available. The importance, therefore, of A-levels is that once the results are known, the tutors can announce decisions finally taken from within the group of well-motivated and committed pre-selected candidates.

The importance of the personal statement on the UCAS form

The personal statement is section 10, the last part of the form but certainly the most important and influential. Most of the UCAS form is a factual summary of what you have achieved but here you have your first chance to give expression, clarity and style to your application and hence bid for a place at veterinary school. Begin by photocopying this page and practising your answer. There is no objection to getting the personal statement typed; indeed it may be wise to do so if your writing is hard to read. An alternative is to use either the Electronic Application Service (EAS) or the internet version, both of which allow you to complete the form on a computer, and email it to UCAS. If either of these are available to you, use them, because your form will be neater, better laid out and easier to read. The software also checks for common mistakes such as missing information, and errors in dates and examination boards. There is also the point that you can usually get more words in the space by typing your answer, but be careful, brevity can often produce a better, more directed, answer!

Research shows that it is a good idea to structure your response. Consider using subheadings to give clarity for the busy admissions tutor.

Make sure that the following points are covered in your personal statement:

- Why do you want to be a veterinary surgeon? There are many possible reasons and this is where your individuality will show.
- Outline your practical experience. Give prominence to the diverse nature of it, the clinics, farms and stables, etc. Mention any interesting cases.
- You like animals, but how do you respond to people? How did you get on with vets, nurses and the customers? Any teamwork experience?
- Give an indication of your career direction, even if it is tentative at this stage. Show that you have thought about the possibilities.
- Any special achievements or responsibilities either connected with animals or with an outside interest?
- List other activities and interests of a social, cultural or sporting kind. Here is your chance to reveal more about yourself as an individual.

Finally, remember to take a copy of section 10 before you pass the completed form to your referee. The copy will serve to refresh your memory before you are called for interviews.

Referee's report

After completion of pages one, two and three of the UCAS form it is ready to be passed, with the completed acknowledgement card and the prescribed fee, to your referee for page four to be completed. Follow the UCAS instructions, do not write anything on page four yourself. It is the responsibility of the referee to post or email the form directly to UCAS. This is usually your headteacher who can draw upon the opinions of the staff and information contained in the school records. However, mature students or graduates for whom school was too long ago for such a reference to be meaningful should approach people who know them well. A good idea is to consider asking someone for whom they have recently worked.

References are an important factor since they provide insight into your character and personality. They can also provide significant confirmation of career aims, achievements and interests. The referee's view of your abilities in terms of analysis, powers of expression and willingness to question things, are the kinds of independent information about you that will have an influence with selectors. Additional information about family circumstances and health problems, which candidates rarely offer about themselves, will also be taken into account.

Table 2 – The following example is illustrative only. It shows the way in which an applicant might structure the personal statement in section 10 of the UCAS form.

---

10 PERSONAL STATEMENT (do **NOT** attach additional pages or stick on additional sheets)

My determination to study Veterinary Medicine has been reinforced by my work experience with both large and small animals. I find working with animals hugely rewarding and I have always had a strong interest in their care and welfare. Veterinary Medicine would give me further opportunities to pursue my interest in science, and apply my knowledge to tackle a wide variety of problems in diagnosis, treatment and research. Veterinary Medicine combines all aspects that I would look for in a vocation, including working closely with people and working as part of a team. Below is a summary of my work experience to date:

3 weeks Hayes Park dairy farm, including calving	1 week Blue Cross
1 week Glades Veterinary Surgery (Small Animal)	2 weeks Forest Stables
1 week Hunters House Veterinary Surgery (Mixed Practice)	1 day Smith's Abattoir
2 weeks Equine Veterinary Practice	3 years Slemans Barn Farm (Stables)
1½ weeks Crocketts Farm (Public) including lambing	1 year Bilbow Stables

At Hayes Park, I was able to take an active role in all aspects of calf husbandry and found the 'hands-on' and practical nature of the work very appealing. Working at the farm also highlighted the difficulty farmers have in balancing commercial and welfare aspects in farming. This was particularly evident during the foot and mouth crisis where it appeared that many of these problems can be due to commercial pressures, such as ever-decreasing market value of livestock. Whilst working at Crocketts Farm I worked with a variety of animals from rabbits and guinea pigs to zebu and llamas. This work also included lambing, often in front of the general public. I frequently had to answer questions about what was happening and explain my actions. This customer aspect of the work was very satisfying. The time I spent in local veterinary practices allowed me to assist and watch both basic and more complex surgical procedures. I found it fascinating being able to watch an endoscopy being carried out on the oesophagus of a horse and I was able to relate my knowledge of biology to what I was seeing. My equine veterinary experience showed me how I could combine my love of horses with a career in veterinary medicine. I also enjoyed participating in the 'Vetsim' and 'Vetsix' courses .

Interests and Responsibilities
Horseriding (I own a 7-year-old gelding and am actively involved in all aspects of his care and schooling); **Duke of Edinburgh** (Achieved the Bronze and Silver awards and currently completing the Gold award); **Manston Drama Club** (local theatre group – I played lead in last production) Music (Grade 4 piano, Grade 5 flute and currently working towards Grade 5 Theory); **School Prefect**.

Following my exams, I have arranged to travel to South Africa for three months. I will spend my time teaching in local primary schools for under-privileged children and working in the Simbari game reserve. The game reserve activities include wildlife veterinary work, game monitoring and assisting with guests at the Game Lodge.

Other supporting documentation

Because work experience in veterinary practices and farms is so important in the selection of applicants for veterinary school, you will be expected to list full details of all such experience. Some veterinary schools will send you a questionnaire asking you to expand on the information you have given about work experience on the UCAS form. Applicants can expect interested veterinary schools to follow up and write on a confidential basis to the veterinary practices and farms where you have worked for additional information about you. This is a good sign as it shows that your application has aroused more than a passing interest.

In essence the veterinary school will ask whether the people you have worked with regard you as a suitable entrant into the veterinary profession. The sorts of things which concern tutors are:

- general enthusiasm;
- ability to express yourself clearly;
- helpfulness;
- practical ability;
- attitude to the animals, to customers and clerical and nursing staff in the practice. (In other words, were you a pleasure to have around?)

So it is clear that the veterinary school can take steps to get hold of additional information about candidates. It is also possible for you to help yourself by taking the initiative to gain documentary support. For example, wait until after you have received your UCAS acknowledgement with your application number, then ask your local vet to write in to the veterinary school(s) of your choice (quoting your reference number) giving details of the five weeks' work which you did with extra detail on any interesting cases with which you were involved. This information will go into your file and is bound to help, especially if the vet is able to say that he or she 'would like to see this person in veterinary school'.

There are exceptions to this arrangement. For instance, the Royal Veterinary College would prefer that copies of all supporting statements, references and case books are brought to your interview rather than sent in advance.

What about mature students?

In view of the extreme competition it is unrealistic for mature students, at say age 25–30 years, to expect special treatment. They must usually expect to satisfy the academic entry requirements in the usual way at one recent sitting and must have a good range of practical experience. However, this requirement has been known to be waived in exceptional cases, such as where there might be a mature student displaying strong motivation coupled with academic ability.

Mature applicants should use section 10 of the UCAS form to set out their qualifications and work experience. Your objective is to signal to the admissions tutors why they should see you. Your extra maturity and practical experience should show here. Photocopy the section and practise expressing yourself in the space provided. If you cannot get all the information on the form make sure you summarise what you want to get across under the main subheadings. Remember it is very important to show why you want to work with animals and to give details of any relevant work experience of a paid or voluntary nature. If you feel that the space in section 10 on the form did not permit you to do full justice to yourself, it's a good idea to prepare a curriculum vitae or further documentation and *wait until you get your UCAS acknowledgement*. The acknowledgement will give you your UCAS application number and you can quote this when you send your additional information direct to the veterinary school.

What to do when rejected

With anywhere between three and five applicants for every place there are inevitably going to be many disappointed candidates. Generally one of the main reasons for rejection is insufficient practical experience, particularly a lack of farm work. If this is true in your own case, the action you could take is to try and remedy the deficiency between the A-level examinations and the publication of the results. All applications are reconsidered after the A-level results are known. If your academic results are satisfactory it may be possible to offer you a place for the subsequent year.

Rejected applicants who have reached the necessary academic standard or have narrowly fallen short should think carefully before turning away from veterinary science, if that is really what they want to do. There are plenty of cases of people who have persisted and gained the extra practical experience that was needed to tip the scales in their favour. Determination to succeed is a quality that is generally recognised and supported. Think carefully before turning away to take another science subject. In most cases such a move will prove to be a decisive career choice. This is because it is not possible to transfer from another science course into veterinary school. Nor is it easy to take veterinary science as a second first degree. This is because graduate applicants have to face stiffer competition and the prospect of having to pay high fees if accepted.

Repeating A-levels

Many unsuccessful candidates decide to do a repeat year and take the examinations again. Before doing this it would be sensible to seek the advice of an admissions tutor. The fact is that not many people doing repeats are made conditional offers unless there are documented extenuating circumstances, such as serious illness. If they are made an offer it will usually be based upon the *second attempt* and the requirement would most likely be raised to achieving grade A in all three subjects. The candidate who may get a repeat offer is one who has narrowly failed to secure a place on the first try and is excellent in all other respects. However, most candidates who reapply have to take their chance in Clearing after a preliminary rejection.

The truth is that the almost overwhelming pressure of demand by highly motivated and well-qualified candidates is taking its toll on the chances of those repeating A-levels. Selection is becoming more stringent, resulting in fewer resitters being successful.

It is possible to improve A-level grades by retaking anything between one and six units, depending on how many times the units have been sat and how close you are to the A-grade boundary. It is often sensible to retake AS units as they are easier than the A2 units. To achieve an A grade at A-level you need to score 480 UMS marks out of 600, and it doesn't matter how the 480 is achieved so it makes sense to gain as many of the 'easier' marks as possible. Your retake strategy will depend on how many extra marks you need, which examination board set your papers (which will determine when resits are available), and how many times

39

you have sat the individual units. Independent sixth form colleges are usually happy to advise students about their options.

26-year-old Nicky is already a graduate. She comes from Liverpool, and is completing her third year of the veterinary science course.

'At a very early age, before I was even nine or ten, I knew that I wanted to be a vet. It's not something I can fully explain. Even as a young girl I wanted a Fisher Price farm rather than any dolls! Looking back it's surprising, especially as I grew up in the city and my family had no farming connections.

'I approached a local vet myself when I was about ten years old. Three years later I was taken on as a kennel maid. Later I gained further contacts from other vets and things just went from there.

'I was a bit of a rebel in the sixth form and didn't do much revision for A-levels and ended up with a B and two Cs, so I couldn't take up my conditional offer from Edinburgh. I then did what seemed a good idea at the time: I took an Animal Physiology and Nutrition degree at Leeds and got a 2.1. I started a PhD but soon realised I was not suited to it. All this time I was asking vet schools if they would accept me. I was shortlisted at London but just missed out and Liverpool declined the first time I asked.

'I knew that I could not give up now and so continued to work with vets whenever I could, especially during holidays. Eventually I think Liverpool took the view that I had proved myself and I was admitted to the course on a self-financing basis since I already had a degree. I am so glad that, at last, I am on the course I've always wanted to do. I enjoy working with animals and I like the lifestyle. This course is leading me towards what I consider to be the best job in the world!'

Richard sat his A-levels last year, and is in his first year studying veterinary science in Scotland. Richard was brought up in London, but his family moved to Essex at the start of his final year of GCSEs. Richard had wanted to be a vet since the age of eleven, when his school went on a visit to London Zoo and were allowed behind the scenes and were given a talk by a vet who worked there. 'We had always had pets at home, including cats, dogs and various small animals and birds. At times, home was like an animal sanctuary as my mother was always looking after neighbours' pets. To be honest, I found them all a bit boring, and it was only the visit to the zoo that made me sit up and realise that being a vet involved more than putting down sick animals or vaccinating them when they were young.'

The change of school disrupted Richard's studies. Having been on target for A and A* grades at his previous school, he only managed to gain two A grades. 'Under the old A-level system I would have been in trouble because I would have been judged only on my GCSE grades and A-level predictions, but mine was the first year to sit AS levels, and I was determined to do well as I knew that if I did, I could show that my GCSE grades were not a true reflection of my ability. I took Biology, Chemistry, Maths and Psychology and got A grades in each one. I then carried on with Biology, Chemistry and Maths and got AAA. I had two interviews, and got an offer from the first one. I was probably overconfident in the second since I already knew I had an offer, and I was surprised to be rejected. Luckily, I got the grades that I needed and so didn't need an insurance offer.'

Richard started getting work experience in the summer following his GCSE examinations. He worked for three weeks on a local farm 'mainly painting fences, but also being able to feed the cattle and help with milking', and spent a further week on another farm near Edinburgh where his uncle lived. 'That is why I decided that I wanted to study in Scotland – not only because I liked the area, but also I thought that I would have an advantage over other applicants since I had worked there.' The following summer, Richard spent two weeks with a vet in a nearby town, mainly concentrating on domestic pets, and a further week with the vet who visited the farm in Scotland. 'I was lucky – my school helped me to organise the first placement with a vet, and my cousin was already shadowing the Scottish vet and she asked him if I could come along. The irony was that I got a place and she didn't! Luckily, she now has an offer for next year but at a different vet school.'

Richard has enjoyed the first year of his studies, but finds some of the work hard. 'The pace is different from A-level, and it is not just a question of learning notes – they want to find out if we understand as well: not like school! Another thing that makes it harder is that my parents are not around to tell me to do my homework every night, and there are lots of opportunities to go out and enjoy life. Still, I think I am just about coping but I know that I'll have to work harder next term.'

COURSE ENTRY REQUIREMENTS

The academic requirements of the six veterinary schools are similar, but there are differences, and it is important that you obtain the most up-to-date information before deciding where to apply.

Information can be found:

- In the university prospectus
- On the university websites (more likely to be up to date)
- *Degree Course Offers*, by Brian Heap
- From the university admissions staff.

Details of all of these can be found at the end of this book.

For A-level students, the selectors will take into account:

- GCSE grades
- AS choices (and, possibly, grades)
- A-level (A2) predictions
- A-level (A2) grades
- Any documented extenuating circumstances that might have affected your performance.

GCSE grades
You will be asked for 'good grades at GCSE'. What does this mean? It means lots of A and A* grades, particularly in the sciences, English and Mathematics. If you did not get good GCSE grades, you can still apply for veterinary science, but your referee should make it clear why you did not achieve the grades that you needed – there may have been circumstances, such as illness, that affected your performance.

AS-levels
The first year of sixth-form study used to be a chance to make the transition from GCSE to A-level and to explore new, more self-directed, ways of studying. The new A-level system – AS-levels in four or five

subjects at the end of the first year, three or four carried on to A2 level the following year – has made life more difficult since lower-sixth students now sit public examinations, the grades from which will feature on the UCAS form, after three terms. Even those universities that state that they will not make offers based on AS grades may take them into account: for example, when faced with two candidates whose academic backgrounds are identical except that one has AAAA at AS-level whilst the other has CCCC, who do you think they would favour? The veterinary schools vary in their policies towards AS-levels. All of them will make offers based on A-levels, usually AAB or AAA, but they may also look at AS grades. Additionally, the choice of AS/A2 subjects is important. For instance, Cambridge is likely to ask for AS Chemistry and two out of Biology, Physics and Mathematics, with at least one of these four taken to the full A-level.

A-levels
The minimum requirement is likely to be at least AAB.

For applicants with Scottish qualifications, it is likely that you will be asked for AAABB or higher in your Highers (SCE/SQA) and CSYS/AH in Chemistry and at least one other science subject. Some veterinary schools like candidates to take a new subject at Higher level if only two CSYS subjects are taken in the sixth year. Highers alone are unlikely to be sufficient.

The **Irish Leaving Certificate** is unlikely to be accepted as equivalent to GCE A-level. This is because studying a wider range of subjects to a lower or less specific level than the UK's A-levels does not meet the need of the veterinary science course requirements. Therefore, this qualification must be offered in combination.

The **International Baccalaureate** is usually acceptable provided that appropriate combinations of subjects are studied. Three subjects are needed at the Higher Level. They must include Chemistry and Biology, together with ideally either or both of Biology, Physics or Mathematics. Grade scores needed: in the Highers are likely to be 7, 7 and 6. If the combination is likely to be different advice should be sought. Similar subject combinations are required by those offering the **European Baccalaureate** with average 8.0 score, to include Chemistry and Biology.

Melanie's parents are both vets, and so she was able to experience the highs and lows of veterinary science from first hand. Her parents were keen for her to follow them, but Melanie was reluctant to do so:

'I felt that they were putting too much pressure on me, and that they were only interested in handing over the family business to me, rather than considering what I wanted to do. Because of this, I did not try very hard in science subjects at GCSE, and chose arts subjects at A-level, probably just to spite them.

'However, when I was working on my UCAS form, I realised that I didn't want to study English or French at university, and that I did, after all, want to be a vet. By then, it was too late to apply because I had the wrong A-levels, so I decided to put in a deferred application, and to study science A-levels in a year after completing my current subjects.

'I got ABB in French, English and History, and then went to a college in London that specialised in one-year A-levels, and studied Biology, Chemistry and Maths. I found this very tough, and there were times when I wanted to give up, but I succeeded in getting interviews and offers from three vet schools, which gave me the incentive to continue.

'Eventually, and after much angst, I got ABC in Biology, Chemistry and Maths respectively. My first choice asked for AAA overall, and rejected me, but my insurance offer was AAB, and I am now in my third year. I have never regretted the decision, and was glad that I swallowed my pride and decided to follow my parents.'

THE INTERVIEW

When the veterinary schools have received the UCAS forms, they will sift through them and decide who to call for interview. Approximately one in three applicants will get an interview, but this can vary from year to year and between universities.

Timing

The timing of interviews can be anywhere from November to March, so some candidates have to wait some time before getting their interview, and because of this timescale some candidates will get a late decision. The Cambridge colleges usually conduct their interviews earlier with the majority taking place in December. This follows on from the earlier start to the application procedure for applicants to the universities of Oxford and Cambridge.

The purpose of the interview

The interview is designed to find out more about you. In particular the interviewers (possibly a panel) will want to satisfy themselves about your motivation and the extent of your commitment to becoming a qualified veterinary surgeon. Have you an appropriate attitude towards animal welfare? Are you reasonably well informed about the implications of embarking on a veterinary career? Are you a mature person possessing a balanced outlook on life? Are they going to be satisfied that you have the ability to last the pace in what is generally acknowledged to be a long and demanding course?

To help them they will have your UCAS form, the headteacher's reference and any supporting statements made by veterinary practitioners or people for whom you have worked. They will already have a good idea of your academic ability or you would not be at the interview in the first place.

Preparation

Experience shows that personal qualities are just as important as academic ability, perhaps more so. The way you come across will be influenced by how confident you are. This doesn't mean being over-confident. Many people believe that they can get through interviews by thinking on their feet, taking each question as it comes. This is an unwise attitude. Good preparation holds the key. By being well informed on a variety of issues you will be able to formulate answers to most questions. There will always be the unexpected question for which no amount of preparation can get you ready, but you can minimise the chance of this happening.

Confidence based on good preparation is the best kind. It is not of the puffed-up variety that can soon be punctured by searching questions. While it is true that the interviewers will want to put you at your ease and will try to make the atmosphere informal and friendly, there is no doubt that for you there will be some tension in the situation. Think positively, this may be no bad thing; many of us perform better when we are 'on our toes'.

Things you can do to prepare

Some schools will be able to offer you a mock interview. Sometimes they can arrange for a person from outside the school to give the interview which can help to give a 'real' feel to it. If you are not sure about whether this facility is available, ask your school careers department. They will be keen to help if they can.

Do you know anyone, student or staff, connected with one of the veterinary schools? If you do, ask for their advice. They may be able to give you an idea of what to expect.

Start your preparation from your copy of section 10 on the UCAS form, ie the personal statement. This is the most important part of your UCAS form and it should tell the interviewers a lot about you as a person, your work experience, your interests and skills. Many of the questions they will ask will be prompted by what you have written in section 10. The questions will most likely begin with those designed to put you at your ease. As the interview proceeds you should expect them to become more searching. Try practising your answers to questions like these:

Question: *Did you have any trouble getting here?*

Comment: This is the sort of friendly question meant to get you started. Don't spend too long on it, take the opportunity to be social, try to get relaxed and smile.

Question: *Have you visited here before?*

Comment: Did you go to the open day? If so, this is the moment to mention the fact. The interviewer will almost certainly follow up and ask what you thought of it. The Faculty probably invested a lot of time and work in preparing it, so go easy on criticism! However, you should be prepared to say what you found was helpful and informative. It is then easier to make an additional constructive criticism. Bear in mind that the interviewers will expect you to have done your homework. If you hope to spend the next five or six years of your life at that institution, you should certainly have made efforts to see whether it is the right place for you. Although your choice is limited to four out of six veterinary schools, you still have a choice to make. If you answer, 'No, but I've heard that you have a good reputation,' you are hardly likely to convince them that you really want to go there. Similarly, answering, 'No, but I think that all of the vet schools are pretty similar,' will not enhance your chances.

Question: *What did you think of our brochure?*

Comment: This is an alternative opening question on which you may have an opinion. Some veterinary schools, like London, have their own brochure; others have their entries in the main prospectus. Be prepared, show that you have at least read it and have an opinion. You could say, 'I thought that it was very informative about the structure of the course, and I particularly liked the case histories of your students – they made me realise that students in a similar situation to me can get a place.' Hopefully, this will lead to a question which will allow you to talk about your work experience.

Question: *How do you think you are doing with your A-levels?*

Comment: This is not a time for false modesty. You would not be having this interview if your school had not predicted good results. You should be sounding optimistic while at the same time indicating that you are working hard. They may also be interested to learn which are your favourite subjects so be ready for a follow-up question along those lines. If you have a good set of AS results, you could mention them at this point. You could also talk about a Biology project which was relevant to veterinary science. As with the two previous examples, your aim should be to steer these rather boring questions towards topic areas that you have prepared and which will show you in the strongest light.

Question: *What do you think of the TV programmes about vets?*

Comment: There are so many of them where do you start? Such programmes could be good or bad for the professional standing of the vet. They make good television, especially when they show the animals and the caring 'honest broker' role of the vet between animals and mankind. On the other hand you could argue that the vet's image is threatened when the programmes degenerate into 'soaps' with a portrayal of young vets which has little to do with their work. In your answer show that you have thought about TV's influence.

Question: *Why do you want to study veterinary science?*

Comment: The direction of the interview can change quite suddenly. Be ready for the switch in questioning; the answer will bring into focus your attitude to animals, the range of your work experience, those important manual skills, and your commitment to all the hard work entailed in studying to become a qualified professional veterinary surgeon admitted to the Register of the Royal College of Veterinary Surgeons. This is an important question and needs a full answer but keep your reply to under two minutes. Practise this. Remember that research findings show that if you exceed two minutes you risk boring your listeners. This is your opportunity, if you have not already done so, to mention your work experience, and to emphasise how your determination to become a vet increased as a result.

Question: *Why do you want to come to this veterinary school?*

Comment: This is a natural follow-up question, so be prepared for it. The answer is personal to you; you may want to go to a new area of the country or you may know the area well because of relatives. Your local vet has recommended this particular veterinary school to you. The reputation of the school may have impressed you because of some particular speciality in which you are also interested. There could be several reasons.

Question: *Tell us something about your work experience with animals.*

Comment: This is one of the big questions of the interview. It would be surprising if the interviewers do not already have feedback from where you have been working. The interviewers will know what happens in a veterinary practice or on a farm, so lists of things that you saw or did will not shed any light onto your suitability for the profession. Instead, concentrate on your reactions to the experience. Did you enjoy it? Were there any interesting or unusual cases that stick in your memory? Does any of your enthusiasm show? Do you indicate any respect and sympathy for the animals? And what about the people – did you get on with them? The key phrases here are, 'For example, when I …' and 'For instance, I was able to …'

Question: *What are the main things you learned from your work experience?*

Comment: This is the typical follow-up question that gives you a chance to summarise and underline your impressions. You could try to indicate the varied nature of your experience, the different types of practice or farm. There is also the business side of working with animals for which you hadn't originally been prepared. Maybe you were astonished at the responsibilities of the veterinary nurses. Be prepared to intrigue your listeners. A related question is, 'From your work experience, what do you think are the qualities necessary to be a successful vet?' Rather than answering, 'Stamina, communication, physical fitness, problem-solving … [and so on]', bring in examples of things that you saw. For example: 'The ability to solve problems. For instance, when I accompanied a vet to a riding school, it was clear that one of the horses was very distressed, but it was unclear why …' and then go on to explain the steps involved in the diagnosis and treatment.

Question: *Have you ever felt frightened of animals?*

Comment: Vets don't like you to be frightened of animals, particularly small ones! However, honesty compels most of us to admit that we have at times and in certain situations felt vulnerable to a kick or bite. Explain the situation and what was said at the time – vets are noted for their humour!

Question: *What do you think of rearing animals for meat?*

Comment: This type of question might be asked because it checks on your motivation. Perhaps you should start by looking at it from the animal viewpoint. Animals should be kept well with good standards of husbandry and eventually slaughtered humanely. Of course, the animal doesn't know the reason for its being slaughtered, but you do. Some of your future clients may be farmers who make their living from supplying meat or poultry – what is your reaction?

Question: *How do you feel about cruelty to animals?*

Comment: With the strong interest in and liking for animals that you would expect from all veterinary students, they will be watching your reaction. This is a question that you should expect and your response, which while putting animal welfare first, should be strong and well reasoned rather than too emotional. What would you do if you thought a farmer was acting in a cruel way to some of his livestock? Go to the police straight away? Talk over the difficulty with a colleague? Threaten the farmer by mentioning that you might bring in the RSPCA? The interviewers are not expecting you to come up with a perfect answer but rather to show that you are capable of coming up with a well-balanced and reasoned solution.

CONTROVERSIAL ISSUES

Most interviews last only 15–20 minutes so there may not be time for questions of a more controversial nature, but nevertheless it may be worth you investing a little thought in how you might sketch out an answer.

Question: *How do you feel about animals being used for medical and veterinary research?*

Comment: You cannot become a veterinary scientist without accepting that you have an obligation to undergo training in all aspects of veterinary science. This must include the use of autopsies on animals, the handling of animal tissues for not only teaching but research and also the use of animals in the teaching programme. Furthermore, every drug available from a pharmacist for human use will have been fully tested. Animals play a large part in these research programmes, so what conclusion do you draw from this? This is an important question as a potential veterinary student who has anti-vivisectionist beliefs and objects to this on conscientious grounds will not be accepted into veterinary school.

Question: *What do you feel about blood sports?*

Comment: This is very much a personal matter. The interviewers may be looking to see whether you can come down on one side or the other while at the same time being able to understand the opposing view. The best way of approaching this is to explain both sides of the argument before giving your own opinion. Make sure that you keep up to date with news stories and new legislation, and avoid 'tabloid' responses. In January 2001, MPs voted to impose a total ban on fox hunting. However, the general election in 2001 meant that the ban was not passed. In March 2002, following debates in the House of Commons and House of Lords, a six month consultation period was announced. The *Guardian* newspaper's website has lots of information to prepare you, whichever way you wish to argue (www.guardianunlimited.co.uk).

Question: *What do you think about keeping animals alive beyond their normal lifespan?*

Comment: In answering this type of question you ought to consider animal welfare. Be alert for the moral dilemma posed. There are reports of dogs fitted with pacemakers which can keep them alive almost indefinitely. If you believe that keeping animals alive beyond when they can have a useful and enjoyable life is wrong you should say so. In general animals eat, sleep and enjoy their lives in that way. By keeping them alive beyond what is natural you can hardly be said to be acting in the interest of the animal's welfare. Would there be circumstances in which a companion animal was essential to the well-being of its owner? Be prepared to discuss these issues rationally. A related question might be asked about the use of antibiotics in animal feed. Make sure that you know why this is done and what dangers this presents.

Question: *Should a vet agree to implement the provisions of the Dangerous Dogs Act?*

Comment: This is a difficult and therefore unlikely question for you to have to face. Show that you are aware that there have been some vicious attacks by certain breeds of unmuzzled dogs on children and adults which led to the Act requiring owners to register this class of dog with the police and keep them muzzled. Controversy arises when the vet might be called upon to destroy, for example, an unmuzzled pit bull terrier *before* it has committed an offence. Is such action contrary to the professional oath of a veterinary surgeon? (Privately many vets are saying that the Act is unworkable.) If you take a view on this you will get credit for at least knowing about the law, whether the interviewer agrees with your conclusion or not.

Question: *What do you know about BSE?*

Comment: Given that there has been enormous publicity about Bovine Spongiform Encephalopathy (BSE), you should certainly be aware of the background to the problem. In 1988, the UK government introduced legislation aimed at stamping out the disease. However, the number of cases continued to rise, reaching a peak in 1993 (over 30,000 confirmed cases). There were about 1000 confirmed cases in 2001. It is thought that BSE was derived from scrapie, a disease that affects sheep. Animal feed containing matter from diseased sheep was then fed to cattle, which caused a variation of scrapie, BSE. It is likely that the disease then spread in two ways: vertical transmission (from the dam to the calf); and from the use of animal feed containing meat from diseased cattle. A variation of the disease, CJD, spread to humans, leading to legislation concerning the age above which cattle could not be sold for human consumption (30 months), the sale of bone-in beef, and animal identification and tracing. The Defra website (www.defra.gov.uk) carries detailed information, and more general articles can be found on the *Independent* newspaper's site (www.independent.co.uk).

CURRENT ISSUES

You must aim to keep up to date with new developments which affect the veterinary profession. The best sources of these are the broadsheet newspapers. As well as the news sections, the health sections contain articles that will be of interest. Your interviewer will want to find out whether you are genuinely interested in the profession, and one way to test this is to investigate your awareness of current issues: after all, if you are planning to devote the next 40 or so years of your life to veterinary science, you ought to be interested in issues that affect the profession. Read a newspaper every day, cut out or photocopy articles of interest, and keep them in a scrapbook so that you can revise before your interview. Other stories that keep cropping up in the newspapers include the issue of badgers and bovine TB, and pet travel schemes. (See following chapter for more information.)

WHY THE INTERVIEW IS IMPORTANT

These are just a few of the possible questions that you might expect at a selection interview for entry to veterinary school. To be called for interview is a positive sign as it indicates that your application is being considered and a good interview can lead to an offer. Another reason for trying to do well at the interview stage is that those candidates whose grades fall just below that required in their conditional offers are always reconsidered. If places are available, a good interview performance could tip the balance in your favour.

Body language and your general appearance and demeanour

A lot could be said about this but it applies to interviews generally. Most candidates will do their best to prepare well for the interview by anticipating likely questions. However, very few candidates realise that the visual impression they are creating will count for much more than their verbal answers to questions. It's a bit like the old saying, 'It's not what you say but the way that you say it'!

Admissions tutors are unlikely to admit that they are going to be influenced by appearance and body language, but they are only human. There is bound to be subjectivity involved. What can you do about it? Try to look your best and try to be as relaxed as possible in what will seem to be a fairly tense situation. Here are a few points to watch.

Body language

When you first enter the room smile and give a firm handshake.

Veterinary schools are friendly places and like to exude informality.

Sit comfortably and reasonably upright, leaning forward slightly. This position makes you look and feel alert. Try not to be so tense that you are crouching forward giving an impression of a panther about to spring. Don't go to the other extreme of leaning back and looking irritatingly self-assured. Where do you put your hands during the interview? Try resting one on top of the other over your lap. Alternatively let each hand rest by your side. It's not a good idea to have your arms folded – it looks as though you are shutting the interviewer out!

Speak clearly and deliberately. Don't rush things. When people are nervous they tend to speed up which makes it harder for the listener. Make eye contact by looking at the questioner. If it is a panel interview let your glance take in others at the table, make them feel that they are included. You should certainly have one or more than one mock interview, which, if possible, should be recorded on video so that you can see how you come across. You will then be able to spot any mannerisms, such as talking with your hand over your mouth or cracking your knuckles, that might distract the interviewers.

Your appearance

Look your best. This does not mean that you should appear like a tailor's dummy. Wear clothes which are smart, not showy, and in which you feel comfortable. Pay attention to details like polishing your shoes and washing your hair.

STUDENT PROFILE

Chris is a Yorkshireman, but all his secondary schooling was on the Wirral. He is about to finish his fifth year of study and qualify as a veterinary surgeon. He is 23 years old, having entered the course straight from school.

'I got interested in becoming a vet when I was about 14. The Herriot books were an influence. I'd always wanted to work outdoors and had wanted to be interested in a job that you could grow into. There was a progressive feel to veterinary science.

'As a family we took our holidays in the country and it was a family friend, a vet, who advised that I needed to get experience. I had about four weeks' experience over weekends and holidays with a vet, attending mostly dairy farms. I did unpaid work gathering in sheep when they were still small. I also helped with dipping sheep and milking cows after a while. At the veterinary practice I was allowed to operate the anaesthetic equipment under supervision. At that stage I didn't really grasp all that was going on, but it was good experience.

'With A-levels I am convinced that it pays to try and finish each syllabus early and then you have several weeks to practise answering questions. Looking back I feel that I took a risk in listing only three veterinary schools plus courses in Pharmacology and Physiology. As it happened I received a conditional offer which I was able to confirm after getting straight A grades. In the event there was no need for all the caution recommended by my school. If I had listed only veterinary schools I could still have opted to enter Clearing if my grades had fallen short of the target.

'On the vet course it has surprised me that there is no course work before exams. I expected lots of essays, but the exams form the assessment. I believe it's only possible to get through a veterinary science course with strong motivation. So I think you must keep clearly in focus what you're going to end up doing. My practical rotations helped me to do this. They included working at the PDSA. It was useful to jam a stethoscope into my ears so that I couldn't hear anyone; it gives you time to think!

'The majority of students here want to go into practice, few want to become specialists. I've already got my first salaried appointment in the north of England plus a house and a car. Vets don't earn enormous sums. My advice to those at school is to talk to the local vets, get to know them and what they do.'

BSE

Bovine Spongiform Encephalopathy (BSE) was first identified in 1986, although it is possible that it had been known about since 1983. It is a neurological disease that affects the brains of cattle, and is similar to scrapie, a disease of sheep that has been known about since the 18th century. In 1988, the government's working party, chaired by Sir Richard Southwood, stated that there was minimal risk to humans since, as scrapie was not known to spread to humans, neither would BSE. It is believed that BSE originated in cattle as a result of the practice of using the remains of diseased sheep as part of high-protein cattle feed in an attempt to increase milk yields. In 1989, the government recommended that specific offals – such as the brain and the spleen – should be discarded rather than allowed to enter the food chain, and that diseased cattle should be incinerated. In the early 1990s, the increased incidence of CJD – a disease similar to BSE that affects humans – caused scientists to look at the possibility that the disease had jumped species. At about the same time, scientists found increasing evidence of transmission between species following experiments involving mice, pigs and cats. By 1993, there were over 800 new cases of BSE a week, despite the ban on animal feed containing specified offals. It became clear that the increase in the cases of CJD was related to the rise in BSE, and that it was likely that millions of infected cattle had been eaten. In 1996, the EU banned the export of cattle, beef and beef products that originated in the UK. In 1997, the government set up a public inquiry, chaired by Lord Phillips. The findings were released in October 2000. Details can be found on the inquiry website (www.bseinquiry.gov.uk/). The total number of cases of BSE in Great Britain since 1986 is estimated to be about 180,000. There were about 1000 new cases in 2002.

The BSE problem raised a number of issues concerning farming and food safety. In retrospect, the decision to allow the remains of diseased animals to be incorporated into animal feed seems to be misguided, at the very least. The problem with BSE is that the infecting agent, the prion (a previously unknown pathogen composed of proteins) was able to survive the treatments used to destroy bacteria and viruses. If any good has come out of the problem, it is that we are now much more aware of food safety. In April 2000, the government established the Food Standards Agency, created to 'protect public health from risks which may arise in connection with the consumption of food, and otherwise to protect the interests of consumers in relation to food'. Although it has been established by the government, it has the independence to publish any advice that it gives the government, avoiding the accusations of cover-ups and secrecy levelled at the government over the BSE affair.

FOOT AND MOUTH DISEASE

The outbreak of foot and mouth disease (FMD) that occurred in February 2001 was the first in the UK for 20 years. The last major outbreak was in 1967, during which about half a million animals were slaughtered. Before the re-emergence of the disease, in a new and highly virulent form, it had been thought that FMD had been eradicated from Western Europe. The latest form of the virus seems to have originated in Asia, and could have been brought into the UK in a number of ways. Something as trivial as a discarded sandwich containing meat from an infected source – brought in to the country by, for example, a tourist – could have been incorporated into pig swill (pig food made from waste food) and then passed on to animals from other farms at a livestock sale. The BSE problem led to greater regulation over abattoirs, which resulted in the closure of many smaller abattoirs. Animals destined for slaughter now have to travel greater distances and the possibility of FMD being passed to other animals is, as a consequence, greater.

The UK was declared foot and mouth free on 14th January 2002, almost a year after the first reported case. More than four million animals, from over 7000 farms, were slaughtered during the period. The last recorded case occurred at the end of September 2001. The official report highlighted the lack of speed with which the government acted and commented on the fact that the understaffed State Veterinary Service was unable effectively to monitor the disease. The disease took a month to diagnose and by the time animal movement was halted, over 20,000 infected sheep had spread the virus across the UK.

A Royal Society report recommended that vaccination – commonly used in a number of countries – should be a weapon in any future outbreaks. Vaccination is unpopular with some meat exporters since it is difficult to distinguish between animals that have been vaccinated and those that have the disease, and for this reason many FMD-free countries ban the import of vaccinated cattle.

FMD is a viral disease that affects cattle, pigs, sheep, goats and deer. Hedgehogs and rats (and elephants!) can also become infected, and people, cats, dogs and game animals can carry infected material. The virus can be transferred by saliva, milk, dung, the breath of infected animals and also can become airborne where it can travel large distances, perhaps as much as 150 miles. A vehicle that has driven through dung from an infected animal can carry the virus to other farms on its tyres. It is more contagious than any other animal disease, and the mortality rate amongst young animals is high.

The role of the veterinary surgeon in a suspected outbreak of foot and mouth disease is not a pleasant one. If the existence of the disease is confirmed, the vet must make arrangements with Defra to ensure that all animals on the farm (and possibly on neighbouring farms) are slaughtered and then incinerated. There is no question of the vet being allowed to try to treat infected animals.

INTENSIVE FARMING

The mainstays of the British diet are meat and dairy products. Although carbohydrates (such as pasta and rice) are providing a greater proportion of our diets than they did ten years ago, we still eat protein in higher quantities than is consumed by our Southern European neighbours. We also demand cheap food. The meat, poultry, dairy and egg industries are faced with a choice – to use technological methods in order to keep the price of their products as cheap as possible, or to allow the animals that they farm to lead more 'natural' lives which would necessarily reduce yields and increase costs. The use of drugs, hormones and chemicals is almost universal in farming (except within the organic farming movement), as are methods to control the movement of livestock by the use of pens, cages or stalls.

The veterinary profession is faced with a number of difficult decisions. It has to balance the need to produce cheap food with its primary aim of maintaining and improving animal welfare. An example of this is the use of antibiotics. Antibiotics are used in farming to treat sick animals. However, they are also used to protect healthy animals against the diseases associated with intensive farming and as growth promoters. The Soil Association reports that about 1225 tons of antibiotics are used each year in the UK, over 60% of which are used for farm animals or by vets. The problem with antibiotics is that bacteria become resistant to them, and overuse of antibiotics in animals has two serious effects:

- Resistant strains of bacteria, such as salmonella and E. coli, can be passed on to humans, causing illness and, in extreme cases, death.
- Bacteria can develop resistance to the drugs that are used to treat serious illness in humans.

Other issues that concern the veterinary profession include:

- The welfare of live farm animals that are exported for slaughter.
- Battery farming of poultry.
- The use of growth hormones.
- Humane killing of farm animals in abattoirs.

The Protection of Animals Act (1911) contains the general law relating to the suffering of animals, and agricultural livestock is also protected by more recent legislation. New regulations came into force in August 2000, incorporating EU law. The regulations cover laying hens, poultry, calves, cattle, pigs and rabbits. Details of the regulations can be found on the Defra website (the address is at the back of this book).

TUBERCULOSIS AND BADGERS

Bovine tuberculosis (bTB) is a serious disease in cattle, and the number of cases is rising. Although the risks of tuberculosis spreading to humans through milk or meat are small, it can be transmitted through other means, particularly to farm workers who have direct contact with the animals. There is uncertainty about the cause of the spread of bTB in cattle, but many people believe that it is passed on by badgers – a protected species. There is widespread support within the farming community for the culling of badgers, but this is opposed by wildlife and conservation groups. In 1998 the government set up a badger-culling trial as well as taking steps to test the carcasses of badgers killed on the roads (about 50,000 every year) in order to try to find out more about the causes of the disease in cattle. However, the results were inconclusive, and the two opposing sides in the argument are still at loggerheads: the fundamental question remains unanswered – is bTB spread from badgers to cattle, from cattle to badgers, or is other wildlife involved?

Bovine TB has been increasing by about 20% a year since 1990, according to Defra. Testing of cattle was suspended during the foot and mouth crisis, but has now resumed.

FOX HUNTING

Most people have a view on the issue of hunting with hounds. On the one hand, there are those who argue that fox hunting is an integral part of rural life; that foxes kill farm animals and therefore need to be controlled; and that thousands of rural jobs will be lost if it is banned. On the other hand, many people believe that it is a cruel and unnecessary way to control foxes, and that the protagonists justify what is merely a barbaric social activity by claiming that it is the most effective way to deal with foxes. The facts are difficult to ascertain. It is claimed that the average duration of a hunt is only 17 minutes, and that the fox is killed by a single bite. Supporters also argue that the total number of people employed as a result of fox hunting is around 16,000, most of whom would then face unemployment since they live and work in rural areas that offer little in the way of jobs. Opponents point out that in some cases, foxes are hunted for hours, and are subjected to multiple agonising injuries before they die. They also argue that the alternatives – shooting by trained marksmen, gassing, snaring or poisoning – are far less cruel in that they do not subject the fox to the trauma of the hunt.

In January 2001, MPs voted to ban outright the practice of hunting with dogs, although the bill has yet to become law.

For opposing sides of the argument, you should investigate the websites hosted by the League Against Cruel Sports (www.league.uk.com/) and the Countryside Alliance (www.countryside-alliance.org/).

ANIMAL TESTING

Almost all of the drugs used to treat us have been tested on animals. Without rigorous and controlled testing there are significant health risks associated with the use of new medicines. In many cases, the long-term or side effects of drugs can be more serious than the illness itself, and testing is therefore essential. Lord Winston, who pioneered in-vitro fertilisation and who more recently found wider publicity through his BBC TV series *The Human Body*, in response to a report by the Lords Select Committee on Science and Technology, was quoted in the *Independent* as saying, 'Perceived pressure may persuade people to go down a route which is not going to promote human welfare. We have a major job – animal research is essential for human welfare. Every drug we use is based on it. Without it those drugs would be unsafe.' The debate on animal testing has become a high profile one in recent months because of the activities of animal rights groups. Although the majority of animal rights groups campaign peacefully, the newspapers have given a good deal of publicity to a number of attacks on research laboratories.

The Home Office reports that, in 1999, over 2.5 million living animals were used in testing procedures. These included 1.6 million mice, 106,000 birds, 6000 dogs and 3000 monkeys. Over 60% of procedures did not involve the use of anaesthetics. Approximately 30% of all testing was aimed at the development of drugs, 20% of all procedures were to investigate toxicity, safety or efficacy of drugs, and about 10% of procedures were related to cancer research. Opponents of animal testing argue that there are alternative methods of testing that do not involve animals. Many of these methods are, they say, also cheaper, quicker and more effective. These include:

- Culture of human cells. This is already used in research into cancer, Parkinson's disease and AIDS.

- Molecular methods, including DNA analysis.
- The use of micro-organisms.
- Computer modelling.
- The use of human volunteers.

The 4000 or so projects licensed by the government are inspected by around 20 Home Office inspectors – a cause for concern amongst vets.

The Royal Society, in a report published in 2001, said that the arrival of genetically modified animals may help to improve animal welfare by reducing disease. Projects underway include research into sheep that are resistant to scrapie. Opponents of genetic modification argue that the creation of disease-resistant animals might be used as an excuse for poor hygiene on farms.

THE COURSES

Given the competitive nature of entry into veterinary school, the idea that there is an element of choice may seem strange. Even when a candidate is fortunate enough to get two or three offers, and has to express a preference, the eventual decision is often based upon things like family connections, the recommendation of the local vet or whether or not the candidate liked the school itself or even the locality on the open day.

Maybe decisions should be made upon more objective data than this, but they seldom are. This may not be a bad thing as decisions made this way often work out quite well. However, although the courses are not vastly different, it is surely sensible for the candidate to be aware of the typical course structure and what is involved. This could be touched upon at interview. Furthermore, a knowledge of some of the differences between courses could play a part in your decision should you get two or more offers.

All the courses leading to a degree in veterinary science have to comply with the requirements of the Royal College of Veterinary Surgeons for recognition under the Veterinary Surgeons Act 1966. This is necessary if the degree is to gain for the holder admission to the Register which confers the legal right to practise veterinary surgery. It follows that the courses are fundamentally similar; most of the slight differences come towards the clinical end of the degree. This is quite a contrast to many other degrees where the differences can be much more marked.

Veterinary courses have a carefully structured and integrated programme with one stage leading logically into the next. This logic is not always apparent to the student who may feel surprised at the amount of theoretical work in the early pre-clinical stage. Later, as you get into the para-clinical and clinical stages, it all begins to make sense. As one final year student commented, 'It's not until the fourth or fifth year that you suddenly realise "so that's why we did that!"'

THE PRE-CLINICAL STAGE

The first two years are pre-clinical and include not only a lot of lectures, but also practicals and tutorials. The normal healthy animal is studied. A basic knowledge of the structure and function of the animal body is essential to an understanding of both health and disease. The scientific foundations are being laid with an integrated study of anatomy and physiology. This study of veterinary biological science is augmented by biochemistry, genetics and animal breeding, as well as some aspects of animal husbandry.

Veterinary anatomy
Deals with the structure of the bodies of animals. This includes the anatomy of locomotion; cellular structure; the development of the body from egg to newborn animal; the study of body tissues such as muscle and bone; and the study of whole organs and systems such as the respiratory and digestive systems. Studying this subject involves anatomical examination of live animals with due emphasis on functional and clinical anatomy. Students spend a lot of their time examining the macroscopic and microscopic structures of the body and its tissue components. One student said, 'We seemed to look through microscopes for hours at various organs and tissues. At the time it was not easy to see the relevance, but later what we had been doing began to make a lot of sense.' There is not only detailed microscopic study of histological sections but also the study of electron micrographs of the cells which make up the different tissues.

Veterinary physiology and biochemistry
Examines how the organs of an animal's body work and their relationship to each other. This is an integral part of the first two years of the course. It is concerned with how the body's control systems work, eg temperature regulation, body fluids, and the nervous and cardiovascular systems. You can expect that your studies will include respiration, energy metabolism, renal and alimentary physiology, endocrinology and reproduction.

Animal husbandry
Extends throughout most courses and introduces the student to various farm livestock and related aspects of animal industries. The kind of

performance expected from the different species and their respective reproductive capacities is investigated. Nutrition and housing of livestock are studied, together with breeding and management. Students learn about the husbandry of domestic animals and some exotic species. Animal husbandry also involves techniques of animal handling. These are important skills for the future veterinary surgeon since the patients will often be less cooperative than those met by their medical counterparts. They may even be much more aggressive than humans!

THE PARA-CLINICAL STAGE

This is sometimes referred to as the second stage. This follows on from the first two years in which normal healthy animals have been studied. Now it is time to undertake studies of disease, the various hereditary and environmental factors responsible, and its treatment. The third year usually sees the study of veterinary pathology introduced (although it sometimes begins in the second year) with parasitology and pharmacology.

Veterinary pathology
Is the scientific study of the causes and nature of various disease processes. This subject is concerned with understanding the structural and functional changes that occur in cells, tissues and organs when there is disease present.

Veterinary parasitology and microbiology
Deals with the multicellular organisms, small and large, which cause diseases and with bacteria, fungi and viruses. All the basic aspects of parasites of veterinary importance are studied. Students also take courses in applied immunology (the body's natural defences).

Veterinary pharmacology
Is the study of the changes produced in animals by drugs (artificial defences against disease). It comprises several different disciplines including pharmacodynamics (the study of the mechanism of the action of drugs and how they affect the body); pharmacokinetics (absorption, distribution, metabolism and excretion of drugs); and therapeutics (the

use of drugs in the prevention and treatment of disease). Some schools introduce this subject in the fourth year.

THE CLINICAL OR FINAL STAGE

The last two years build on the earlier years, with food hygiene being introduced while the study of pharmacology is deepened. The meaning of the phrase 'integrated course' now becomes apparent as all the disciplines come together. Medicine, surgery and the diseases of reproduction are taught by clinical specialists in the final stages of the course which is largely practical. More time is spent at the school's veterinary field station. In some cases you can expect to live in at the field station in your final year. Much of the study will be in small groups. In some cases you will be allowed to pursue particular interests. However, the main focus will be on diagnosis and treatment by medical or surgical means necessary for the prevention, diagnosis and treatment of disease and accidental injury in a wide range of species.

Some of the practical skills used in the clinical stage

There are many important practical skills that students have to learn in the final clinical period. One of these is to be able to examine the contents of the abdomen through the wall of the rectum without harming the animal or infecting themselves.

They can also learn to use an ultrasound probe to examine, for example, the ovaries. Another use of ultrasound is to listen to the foetal heart sounds of a pregnant sow and the blood flow. Ultrasound can also assist in carrying out an examination of a horse's fetlock.

Students, like the vets they hope to become, can be called out in the middle of the night to a difficult calving. If a cow can't give birth naturally, the student can help with a caesarian operation. Using a local anaesthetic allows the operation to take place with the cow standing which makes the process easier to manage. Practical skill is important with foaling. It is best if this takes place quickly because it is less stressful for the foal. Students are taught that all that is needed is a gentle but firm pull. Final-year students can assist with the lambing, even the birth of twin lambs.

There are many examples too numerous to mention. The use of general anaesthetic can extend from a full range of horse treatments to vasectomising a ram. Many other techniques are taught. Students can, for example, look at images of the nasal passages of a horse and see the nasal discharge from a guttural pouch infection. Another example is learning the right way to trim a cow's foot. All animals can suffer problems with their legs or feet.

The experienced veterinary surgeon has to have the skill and the confidence to be able to remove a cyst from a sheep's brain without causing a rupture. No wonder then that it is at this final clinical stage that the student finds that all the earlier preparation comes together and makes sense as clinical problem after problem requires you to think and reason from basic scientific principles.

Examples like these do convey the varied nature of the veterinary surgeon's work, but it is as well to remember that in addition to the physician side of the job there is a lot of routine 'dirty' work. Students have, for example, to help maintain cleanliness in the stables and enclosures of the field station. In due course, when they become working vets, they may at some stage spend time, on a cold wet day, tramping round a muddy farmyard carrying out blood testing of hundreds of cattle.

This brief summary of some of the clinical work encountered on the courses should not lead students to believe that this corresponds to a job description.

EXTRA-MURAL ROTATIONS (EMR)

This is sometimes called 'seeing practice' and the time is divided between farming work and experience in veterinary practice. Students are required during the first two years to complete 10–12 weeks of livestock husbandry, depending on which school they attend. The students usually arrange this experience themselves to take place during their vacations, and on the whole they do not seem to have too much difficulty.

Veterinary schools have lists of contacts that can be made in their own area. A modest amount of pay can be arranged between student and farmer. During the third, fourth and final clinical years students must complete approximately 26 weeks of 'seeing' veterinary practice. This will be mainly with veterinary surgeons in 'mixed' general practice, with much shorter periods in, for example, laboratory diagnostic procedures and one or two weeks in an abattoir. Casebooks have to be kept and presented at the final examination.

NOTES ON THE COURSES

Bristol

An interesting feature of the course at the University of Bristol is that in the pre-clinical departments they teach science, medical and dental students alongside the vets. It is claimed that this encourages cross-fertilisation of ideas and access to the latest research findings in other scientific fields. **Assessment:** This is by examination in January and June each year. **Resits:** There is a chance to resit all or part of the examination in September if the required standard is not reached in June. **Intercalation:** It is possible to interrupt your studies for a year at the end of the second or third year in order to gain additional training for a BSc degree in, for example, Biochemistry, Microbiology, Pathology, Pharmacology and Zoology. **Clinical training:** The Clinical Veterinary School is at Langford in the Mendip Hills, about 13 miles out of Bristol. Extra-mural experience abroad is not allowed at Bristol. There is a government veterinary investigation centre nearby.

Cambridge

This is the smallest of the veterinary schools. The course extends over six years and is divided equally between the pre-clinical and clinical parts. The first two years are concerned with the basic medical and veterinary sciences, between which there is much common ground at this early stage, bringing you into contact with students from other disciplines. There are also more applied courses in Farm Animal Husbandry and Preparing for the Veterinary Profession. For the third year you can elect to study in depth a subject of your own choice from a wide range of options, leading to the award of the BA (Hons) degree at the end of year three, the additional year. The flexibility of the tripos system is one of its most attractive features.

Clinical training: The clinical course is taught in the Department of Clinical Veterinary Medicine on Madingley Road, about two miles from the city centre. The emphasis is on small group practical teaching. The final year is largely lecture free with 'hands-on' experience and a period of elective study. The Farm Animal Practice provides first opinion clinical services to surrounding farms including the University Dairy Farm just a few miles away. A new Farm Animal Referral centre will open in late 2002. Advantage is also taken of the nearby RSPCA clinic, specialist equine practices in and around Newmarket and the Animal Health Trust Centre. A small-animal practice in the centre of Cambridge provides first opinion cases for teaching. New facilities are now complete for Equine work and a new Small Animal Surgical Suite is nearing completion.

Edinburgh

Long established and one of the larger veterinary schools, the Royal (Dick) School of Veterinary Studies can trace its origins back to 1823. The school is now part of the College of Medicine and Veterinary Medicine. Traditional boundaries between subjects have been reduced. Most of the preclinical training is at Summerhall, close to the city centre. Formal teaching is completed in four years, with the final devoted to clinical experience. **Assessment:** Half assessment is continuous, the balance is by examination and practicals. **Resits:** There is a chance to resit the examinations in September if this is necessary. **Intercalation:** It is possible for students to interrupt their studies at the end of years two, three or five to take a BSc (VetSc) degree in one of the following honours schools: Biochemistry, Neuroscience, Virology, Pathology or Preclinical Sciences. Also being introduced is a one-year MSc by research after the third year of studies and the possibility of doing an intercalated three-year PhD during the course of studies. **Clinical training:** This takes place at the Easter Bush Veterinary Centre, six miles south of the city. Here are situated the college farm which is attached to the University's School of Agriculture, the Large Animal Practice, Equine and Food Animal Hospitals and the new Small Animal Hospital. The Centre for Tropical Veterinary Medicine forms part of the school. The BBSRC's Moredun Research Institute, the Roslin Institute and a veterinary investigation centre are situated nearby.

Glasgow

One of the larger schools, founded in 1862. The school has the unique advantage of being situated on a single site at Garscube, four miles to the north west of Glasgow. Some pre-clinical teaching is held at the main university campus near to the city centre, which enables students to benefit from the opportunities at both sites. **Resits:** These can take place in September of each year. A second failure may result in repeating a year; normally this is only possible for one year of the course. **Intercalation:** It is possible at the end of year three to study for a one-year BSc (VetSc) Honours before starting the clinical training. Eight subjects are available. A two-year intercalated BSc Honours degree at the end of either years two or three is another possibility. **Clinical training:** Glasgow was the first school to introduce the lecture-free final year. This was done in order to maximise the opportunities for small group clinical teaching around live animal cases. This takes place at the Faculty's busy referral hospital and through extra-mural study undertaken in practices and other veterinary institutions in the UK and overseas.

Liverpool

The university was the first to establish a veterinary degree. The Faculty of Veterinary Science will be celebrating its centenary in 2004. There are two degree courses leading to BVSc MRCVS – the D100 which is a 5-year course and the D101 which is 6 years incorporating an intercalated BSc. The options for intercalating include a BSc in Conservation Medicine. This course is also offered to students from other veterinary schools. In 2001 the Faculty also introduced a 3-year Honours BSc course in Bioveterinary Science. Teaching on this course is shared between the Faculty of Veterinary Science and the School of Biological Sciences. Veterinary students spend the first three years of the course on campus in Liverpool studying pre-clinical and para-clinical subjects. The course is modularised. During the fourth and final years, the students are based at Leahurst, the teaching hospital on the Wirral peninsula 12 miles away. This has excellent facilities for equine and livestock cases. The Small Animal Hospital is currently sited at Liverpool. A new referral Small Animal Hospital is planned for Leahurst, although first opinion work will continue at Liverpool. There are two separate practices operating out of Leahurst, serving the large local equine population and the agricultural sector. Farm visits and investigations extend to the sheep farming areas of North Wales and the dairy farms of Cheshire and Lancashire. Horses are referred from all areas of northern England, particularly colic, skin tumour and orthopaedic conditions. Leahurst is in close proximity to Chester Zoo and there is a strong interest in wildlife diseases and animal behaviour.

London

The Royal Veterinary College, based in Camden, is the oldest (founded in 1791) and largest of the six UK veterinary schools. After completing the core course each student at the start of the final year selects one of a group of elective subjects to study in greater depth and receives extra tuition to prepare for an examination and the presentation of a 5000 word report as a part of the final examination. **Resits:** This is possible should it be necessary. **Intercalation:** This is available after completion of the first BVetMed Part 2 at the end of year two or after completion of the second BVetMed at the end of year three. Students are able to attend courses offered by medical and science faculties of other institutions within the University of London leading to the award of a BSc. **Clinical training:** The para-clinical and clinical courses extend over years three to five and are based mainly north of London at Hawkshead, Hertfordshire. The College has its own farm at nearby Boltons Park. In addition to the large-animal practice there is the small-animal referral centre at the Queen Mother Hospital, another part of the Hawkshead Campus near Potters Bar. Student study groups also have the chance to take part in the work of the Beaumont Animals' Hospital in Camden dealing with referral small animal medicine and surgery. During the course 38 weeks of extra-mural study must be carried out. It is possible for some of this to be undertaken overseas.

All of the courses aim to produce a graduate with sufficient breadth and depth of knowledge that he or she will be able to adapt to the changing demands of the profession over the 40 years or so of working life.

Table 3 – Undergraduate student numbers 2001/2002

Veterinary School	1 Admissions to veterinary courses (UK students)			2 Those who are already graduates on entry	3 EU and overseas students			4 Those taking an intercalated science course
	M	F	T		M	F	T	
Bristol	30	59	89	5	1	6	7	11
Cambridge	19	54	73	6	0	1	1	62
Edinburgh	24	74	98	30	2	6	8	5
Glasgow	25	57	82	7	2	9	11	2
Liverpool	26	67	93	16	1	3	4	8
London	29	117	146	2	8	13	21	15
TOTALS	153	428	581	66	14	38	52	103

Acknowledgement: Extract from *Royal College of Veterinary Surgeons Annual Report 2002*

FINANCE

Once you arrive in veterinary school you will want at least to avoid the worry of getting too deeply into debt. It is, of course, true that money is a problem for all students and not least with vets who have additional expenses connected with their course. These extra costs can be summarised as being mainly travel expenses, clothing, books and equipment. Vet students are also limited regarding the opportunities they have to earn extra money during vacations due to the extra-mural rotations spent gaining prescribed experience in veterinary practice as part of their training. Students believe that sixth-formers and others approaching veterinary school should be forewarned and prepared to cope with the money side of being a vet student.

First-year expenditure for vets is particularly high and can easily exceed £6000 for those living away from home.

A significant item is the means-tested contribution to tuition fees. According to government sources less than half the student population will have to pay the maximum permitted fee.

The figures estimated in Table 4 will vary according to the student vet's lifestyle and the costs surrounding each veterinary school. The first year is particularly difficult as there are a lot of startup costs to be absorbed. So far as finance is concerned, the home-based student is the only one likely to avoid going into debt. The second year is not quite so expensive. By this time students are learning to make economies and the course demands in textbooks may not be so great. However, the apparent saving on moving away from halls into self-catering accommodation could prove deceptive unless your catering and housekeeping ability is good.

Income

To counterbalance these levels of expenditure the main financial support will come from student loans and bank overdrafts. There are no known sources of sponsorship for undergraduate veterinary students. However, the student loans are not means-tested and you can draw up to the maximum allowed. In addition there are hardship loans and Access Funds for those who find themselves in serious financial difficulties.

No student loan repayments have to be made until after you have finished or left the course. Even then you will not make repayments if your income is below what is called the 'threshold level'. This level is reviewed and set each year by the government.

Table 4 – Expenditure estimate in pre-clinical years
(Note: this is estimated in November 2002 and is intended only as a guide.)

First year	London	Away	Home
Course Fee (max)	£1100	£1100	£1100
Overalls	£45	£30	£30
Lab coats	£40	£25	£25
Wellies	£25	£25	£25
Course notes	£65	£65	£65
Textbooks	£260	£260	£260
Travel costs	£350	£300	£300
EMS travel costs	£260	£240	£240
StudentVet sub	£50	£50	£50
Social events	£1000	£1000	£800
Accommodation	£3300	£2900	*
Total estimated cost	£6495	£5995	£2895

Hints and tips

- Avoid buying lots of kit or textbooks in advance. When you get to the course you may find some discounts available. Second-hand textbooks may be for sale, although many veterinary students prefer to keep their textbooks for use in their working lives. Try medical students as well for second-hand textbooks.
- Check for student travel concessions, get advice on the best offer on the regular trips that you will have to make.
- It is a good idea to apply for the student loan early on as it takes some time for the loan to be processed. You can also make contact with the bank about that overdraft facility they promoted to you when they sought your custom.

- Vet students work hard and like to play hard as well. Set yourself a limit on how much you are prepared to spend each term. Remember the more partying the worse your bank account will look. Perhaps you will go to the annual vet ball. If you do, why not consider hiring the gear? By all means join the Association of Veterinary Students (AVS), but do you want to attend the congress or go on sports weekends? They all cost money.
- Easter is a time when it is possible for students to augment their income. Once you have gained experience with your first lambing, students say that it is possible, if you are lucky, to make up to £300 per week. This is very hard work involving twelve hours a day, for seven days a week, for a minimum of three weeks. But it will certainly improve the look of your bank account – and give valuable experience.

How to keep running totals

One final thought is that it helps enormously if you know how you are doing week by week. Keep a cash book with your income divided into termly income and split into monthly amounts on one side of the book. On the other side enter your corresponding monthly expenditure, including all items from cash for entertainments to rent and utility bills. At the end of each month you can bring the balance forward and see how you are doing. It is surprising how many students overlook this simple precaution.

CAREER PATHS

There may be hidden expenses in training to be a vet but at least you can reflect, with some optimism, that a degree in veterinary science is going to result in a professional qualification and a job. The vast majority of veterinary surgeons, well over 80% of the total at work, are in practice in the UK. There is currently a real shortage of vets. A glance through the pages of the *Veterinary Record* will confirm the strong demand for the newly qualified vet to go into practice. The universities' first destination statistics show that very nearly all students begin their careers in practice but such is the great variety of opportunity in this profession that career change and divergence can and do occur. Graduates are also employed in the government service dealing with investigation, control and eradication of diseases. There are also opportunities for veterinary scientists to become engaged in university teaching and research establishments at home and abroad.

WORKING IN PRACTICE

Should you start in general practice there is the chance to move into different types of practice.

The trend is towards the small-animal practice. There are also more horses – now seen as not just a companion animal but also an important part of the growing leisure industry.

It is clear that the mainly farm animal practice is seeing a dramatic fall in business and is having to diversify. This trend, evident over the last 20–30 years, is accelerating dramatically for a variety of reasons – the uneconomic structure of much of the farm economy and the tendency for farmers to treat simple problems themselves being the most significant factors. Even mixed practices dealing with farm animals as well as small companion animals like cats and dogs are becoming less common.

The size of practices varies a great deal. Some practices are small, the average size is three or four vets working together, while a few are much larger. Some are incredibly busy, others equally hardworking may manage to convey a less rushed atmosphere.

New trend

Membership of the EU has brought a new source of income into general practice. This comes about through increased certification required in the interests of safeguarding public health. Every abattoir has to have an official veterinary surgeon to see that it operates hygienically and that slaughtering is humane. Full-time vets are appointed to the Defra's Meat Hygiene Service. Every port and airport has to have a veterinary surgeon available. No wonder vets are in short supply.

Women in the profession

It's a fact that over twice as many women are admitted to veterinary science courses as men (see Table 3). They comprise about one-third of all the vets in the country and are making a major contribution to animal welfare and the safeguarding of public health. However, in career terms women form only one in five of the sole principals in general practice. Two explanations have been suggested. One is that the statistic reflects past intakes into the profession and this is changing. Another is that whereas women are in the majority at age 30 or younger, they only comprise one in ten of those aged 50 or over. This suggests that they leave the profession early for child rearing and family responsibilities and do not always return. The figures also hint that they are slightly more inclined than their male colleagues to work in the public sector.

Specialisation

There is a growing trend towards specialisation within practices. According to the RCVS 1998 Manpower Survey 80% of vets in general practice spend over half their time with one type of animal. Nearly half of those in general practice spend all their time on small animals. Areas of specialisation include cattle, horses or household pets or even exotics. It can be more sophisticated than that such as combining equine care with lameness in all animals. Dermatology, soft tissues and cardiology are examples of the kinds of specialisation which are seen as helpful to clients. It is possible for postgraduate specialist qualifications to be obtained under the Royal College of Veterinary Surgeons' specialist certificate and diploma examinations.

Table 5 – Numbers and Distribution of the Profession who are economically active

	2002	2001	% change 2001–2002
General Practice	11549	11007	+5%
Government Service	18	19	–5%
Defra	399	401	–0.5%
Food Standards Agency	12	14	–14%
Meat Hygiene Service	49	55	–11%
Ministry of Defence	39	43	–9%
Dept of Agriculture (N. Ireland)	146	137	+7%
Scottish Agricultural College	37	39	–5%
Universities	569	566	+0.5%
Research Councils	27	32	–16%
Industry and Commerce	286	295	–3%
Charities	342	352	–3%
Other	13	13	–
Totals	13486	12973	+4%

Acknowledgement: *Royal College of Veterinary Surgeons Annual Report 2002*

Dealing with people

Being in veterinary practice means that you are running a business. For example, today's vets have to be familiar with computer records on health and production and know how to interpret them, but there is a more important factor. Vets have to be customer-oriented and students soon pick this up. 'The way we approach people is crucial, it's our bread and butter,' remarked one vet. 'It's the same on the telephone. We make a point of being cheerful and reassuring with a few words of advice until we can get there.' This aspect of practice is now so important that some practices are hiring a manager to run the administrative side and help to train reception staff. Most courses now make some attempt to introduce the student to the economics of running a practice, although as one vet commented wryly, 'Few will think of bookkeeping!'

Professional approach

With increasing professionalism and rising customer expectations goes higher overheads. A student at school may not realise the significance of all the things they see in a modern surgery. Look around and first note the condition of the waiting area. It should be comfortable and clean. The kennels should be of good quality and there will most likely be a separate preparation room. Notice all the new equipment, a far cry from the more primitive era described in the Herriot books. It is quite likely that there will be anaesthetic and blood pressure monitoring equipment, radiography, ultrasound and Doppler ultrasound, endoscopy units, orthopaedic instrumentation, operating microscopes, and laser equipment for cataract surgery. To equip a modern veterinary surgery requires a considerable capital sum and so most newly qualified vets will start their working life by going into practice with other vets. Some will aspire to and attain a partnership after two or three moves, a few will, after gaining experience over three or four years, branch out on their own. Another minority moving in other career directions will have more significance than their numbers suggest.

TEACHING AND RESEARCH

A qualification in veterinary science is more than a licence to practise. It can also open up opportunities for those interested in university teaching and research at home and overseas. In addition to clinical research work, some veterinary surgeons undergo further postgraduate training in the biological sciences. Specialisation is possible in physiology, pathology, microbiology, nutrition, genetics and statistics. Veterinary scientists are not exclusively found to be working in institutions concerned with animal health and disease; they can also be found working in natural science laboratories, medical schools and medical research institutes. The opportunities are there for young veterinary surgeons attracted by a research career.

The veterinary schools provide referral hospitals to which veterinary surgeons can refer cases needing more specialised treatment. For example, recent success in the treatment of equine colic has stemmed from early recognition and referral of appropriate cases allied to developments in anaesthesia and monitoring, improved surgical techniques and suture materials plus better post-operative care. Good teamwork between the referring practitioner and the university specialists plays a big part.

Veterinary graduates are employed as research scientists by Defra, the Biotechnology and Biological Sciences Research Council, the Animal Health Trust, and in pharmaceutical and other industrial research organisations.

THE GOVERNMENT

Most of the veterinary surgeons employed by Defra work in either the Meat Hygiene Service, the Veterinary Field Service or the Veterinary Investigation Service. Field officers have a wide range of responsibilities which include the control of major epidemic diseases of farm animals, matters of consumer protection largely in relation to meat hygiene, the control of import and export of animals and the operation of health schemes.

The Veterinary Investigation Service comprises officers who are based in laboratories known as veterinary investigation centres (VICs). Their job is to operate and support control schemes in the interests of public health, to monitor developments and give early warning of any disease problems or dangers to the safety of the food chain. They also provide practising vets with a chargeable diagnostic service. The Central Veterinary Laboratory (CVL) at Weybridge employs veterinary surgeons who carry out research and support for various field activities. The Veterinary Medicines Directorate (VMD) deals with the licensing of drugs.

OTHER CAREER PATHS

Veterinary scientists are needed by the Army. Their duties arise in the Royal Army Veterinary Corps where they care for service animals, mostly working dogs and horses used for ceremonial purposes. They also have public health responsibilities and opportunities for research or postgraduate study. Those recruited join as Army captains for a four-year Short Service Commission, but this may be altered to a Regular Commission on application.

Some veterinary surgeons prefer to work for animal welfare societies, such as the RSPCA, PDSA and Blue Cross. Others work as inspectors for the Home Office.

SUMMING UP

Many students are interested in becoming veterinary surgeons. For some it will remain a pipedream either because they lack the ability or skill, or because their ideas are not rooted in reality. However, there are real opportunities for those who are motivated and determined to reach their goal. The competition is severe but not impossible and students should be encouraged to explore the veterinary option early. They must do this by seeking practical experience. As one vet put it, 'See a farm, get your wellies dirty, experience some blood and gore, and see that the life of a vet is not all about cuddly puppies!' This will test their resolve and suitability.

The demand for veterinary services and research-related activities is strong and is increasing. Market forces do dictate, but funding limitations on the number of places in veterinary schools imposed by the Higher Education Funding Councils are a controlling factor. Nevertheless, the profession of veterinary surgeon retains its popularity among young people. It is not because of the money, the car or accommodation, which is often next to the practice ready for instant call-outs! Nor can long hours be the attraction; the provision of a 24-hour service to the public is mandatory. Rather it is probably the sense that here is a way of life rather than a job.

Is being a veterinary surgeon a unique career?

Consider for a moment that the vet has to be a GP with numerous skills and specialisms. Most practitioners are self-employed with wide variations in income, depending upon the type of practice and location. Yet they must make a big capital investment in the latest equipment as

81

veterinary medicine becomes increasingly technical. In the UK there is no state funding for veterinary practice equivalent to the NHS. All the funding comes from the clients. Yet the vets do not want finance to take over. It is still a caring profession that does not always charge what it should, for example, for compassionate reasons. It is a profession facing immense changes and so it is not surprising that a new career is emerging, that of practice manager. A sensible appointment of a professional manager allows the vets to concentrate on what they do best, dealing with the customers and their animals.

An experienced vet, operating a mixed practice on the Wirral, put the unique qualities of being a vet this way: 'I think people respect what we do. Every Friday a lady brings us a chocolate cake. It's little things like this that make you feel appreciated.' A vet is many things, skilled surgeon, business manager, counsellor and confidant. They know that for their customers the animals are often the most important thing in their lives. They have tremendous responsibility for the animals, whether in sickness or in health, and when all other options have failed they have the authority and power vested in them by law to take the animal's life. They devote their lives to animal welfare but it is not based on sentimentality. Find out if it's the life for you and if it is, *go for it*.

STUDENT PROFILE

It is now over eight years since Joanne qualified as a veterinary surgeon, having studied at Liverpool. Today she is 32, married and working in a mixed practice, dealing with farm animals, horses and small animals in her native Cheshire. 'Immediately after you qualify you discover that you have a steep learning curve, there is so much still to learn.' Much of the stress of being a young veterinary surgeon is in learning how to communicate clearly and calmly with the owners, as well as learning about the many animals presented to you.

More women are becoming vets and I wondered if she had experienced an acceptance problem? She had met some more traditionally minded clients who might say things like, 'This is no job for a woman! We can't ask you to do this!' But, adds Joanne, 'you gain acceptance when they see you are finding alternative ways of coping with some of the more physical aspects of the job.'

In veterinary work the unexpected often confronts you, emergencies occurring, such as horses with colic, cows needing assistance calving, road accidents etc, so the mixed practitioner needs to be flexible and versatile. For example, small-animal emergencies can arise needing blood tests and X-rays, in which case the vet becomes a clinical detective, putting together all the facts before drawing conclusions. In a practice of several vets each may have some specialist area of expertise which colleagues can draw on. To help the vet keep up to date there is training through CPD (Continuing Professional Development) and Joanne takes full advantage of this, attending the British Small Animal Veterinary Association Congress every year. The vets try to avoid duplicating each other's course attendances: this is not difficult because, Joanne says, 'There are plenty of courses and meetings from which to choose.'

Joanne enjoys her work. Asked why, she lists dealing with the animals, the problem solving, the outdoors side to the work and the relationships forged with her clients. The last is very important. In Joanne's experience the ability to communicate clearly with the owner is extremely important.

If she were to offer advice to sixth formers it would be: 'If you don't like people you will not be able to do this job and never even think of this job if you want regular hours.' You have to be willing to take on duty at night and at weekends. Her two dislikes are not surprisingly the unsocial hours and that although she enjoys her contact with clients and gets on well with almost all of them, there are some, as in any job, who can be more difficult to deal with, requiring tact and patience even at the end of a long working day!

Joanne began making enquiries about becoming a vet at the age of 14. It all started with weekend work which included experiencing kennels, a dairy farm and riding stables. Joanne is unsure about her future career direction. She thinks she will continue in general practice which she so much enjoys. At present, in common with all assistant vets, she holds a salaried position in the practice. Eventually it may be possible to buy into a partnership; many assistants do this. (Today about half of the vets in general practice in the UK own a stake in their practice.)

APPENDIX: CONTACTS AND FURTHER INFORMATION

Veterinary schools in the UK

BRISTOL

The Veterinary Admissions Office
University of Bristol
Senate House
Tyndall Avenue
Bristol BS8 1TH
Tel: 0117 928 7679 (direct)
Email: admissions@bris.ac.uk
Website: www.bris.ac.uk

CAMBRIDGE

Veterinary Admission Enquiries Adviser
Department of Clinical Veterinary Medicine
University of Cambridge
Madingley Road
Cambridge CB3 0ES
Tel: 01223 330811
Email: application.advice@vet.cam.ac.uk
Website: www.vet.cam.ac.uk

EDINBURGH

The Admissions Officer
Faculty of Veterinary Medicine
Royal (Dick) School of Veterinary Studies
University of Edinburgh
Summerhall
Edinburgh EH9 1QH
Tel: 0131 650 6138 (direct)
Email: vetug@ed.ac.uk
Website: www.vet.ed.ac.uk

GLASGOW

The Secretary
Admissions Committee
Veterinary School
University of Glasgow
Bearsden Road
Bearsden
Glasgow G61 1QH
Tel: 0141 330 5705 (direct)
Email: J.Wason@vet.gla.ac.uk
Website: www.gla.ac.uk/Admissions

LIVERPOOL

The Admissions Sub-Dean
Faculty of Veterinary Science
The University of Liverpool
Liverpool L69 7ZJ
Tel: 0151 794 4281
Email: vetadmit@liv.ac.uk
Website: www.liv.ac.uk/vets

LONDON

The Registry
The Royal Veterinary College
University of London
Royal College Street
London NW1 0UT
Tel: 020 7468 5148/9 (direct)
Email: registry@rvc.ac.uk
Website: www.rvc.ac.uk

Other contacts and sources of information

The Royal College of Veterinary Surgeons, Belgravia House,
62-64 Horseferry Road, London SW1P 2AF; Tel: 020 7222 2001
Email: education@rcvs.org.uk; Website: www.rcvs.org.uk

Advice for qualified veterinary surgeons from outside the UK who wish to practise in the UK can be found on the RCVS website: www.rcvs.org.uk/vet_surgeons/members/

A summary of the procedures is provided on the website that accompanies this book: www.mpw.co.uk/getintomed

British Veterinary Association – the national representative body for the British veterinary profession. www.bva.co.uk

Society of Practising Veterinary Surgeons – provides advice to veterinary surgeons. www.spvs.org.uk

British Equine Veterinary Association. www.beva.org.uk

The Blue Cross. www.thebluecross.org.uk

People's Dispensary for Sick Animals. www.pdsa.org.uk

Vetsonline – on-line database and resource. www.vetsonline.com

Vetweb – Information network for veterinary professionals with good links to other sites. www.vetweb.co.uk

St George's University, Grenada, WI. Tel: 0800 169 9061
Website: www.sgu.edu

Department for Environment, Food and Rural Affairs (Defra)
Website www.defra.gov.uk

CRAC Degree Course Guide – Veterinary Science – This should be available in most school careers libraries; if not it can be purchased for £7.50 (inc p&p) from: Hobsons: www.hobsons.com

You and Your Vet Popular pet care magazine published quarterly in the interests of companion animals and their owners by the British Veterinary Association: Animal Welfare Foundation (BVA: AWF), and available exclusively from most veterinary practices. It has many useful addresses and can give you a feel of what concerns pet owners and vets.

University and College Entrance: The Official Guide The latest edition is normally published in June and is usually available in school and public reference libraries. Available from www.careers-portal.co.uk

UCAS Handbook: How to apply for admission to a university Published in June free of charge and normally available in schools. Alternatively write for your copy to UCAS, Rosehill, New Barn Lane, Cheltenham, Gloucestershire GL52 3LZ; Tel: 01242 223707
Email: app.reg@ucas.com

VETSIX Two-day conference organised by the Workshop University Conferences for interested sixthformers and held annually at Nottingham. www.workshop-uk.com

VetCam Two-day residential 'Introduction to Veterinary Science in Cambridge' course held in March. Contact Mrs Jill Armstrong: 01223 330811.

Student Loans – A Guide to Applying (Free) Student Loans Co., 100 Bothwell Street, Glasgow G2 7JD; Website: www.slc.co.uk

Financial Support for Students DfES; Tel 0870 000 2288; Website: www.dfes.gov.uk/studentsupport

The Student Book, Klaus Boehm and Jenny Lees-Spalding, £16.99; Trotman; www.careers-portal.co.uk

Students Money Mattters, Gwenda Thomas, £12.99, Trotman; www.careers-portal.co.uk

Degree Course Offers, Brian Heap, £24.99, Trotman; www.careers-portal.co.uk